Table of Contents

Practice Test #1 ....
  Practice Questions 4
  Answers and Explanations 33
Practice Test #2 57
  Practice Questions 57
  Answers and Explanations 82

Practice Test #1

Practice Questions

1. Which of the following is not routinely included as part of a diagnostic work-up for colorectal cancer?
    a. Barium enema
    b. Colonoscopy
    c. Bone marrow biopsy
    d. Carcinoembryonic antigen (CEA)

2. You are a registered nurse working in an outpatient infusion center and have begun administration of paclitaxel on a newly-diagnosed breast cancer patient. The patient mentions that she is feeling flushed and shows you a small hive on her left cheek. Your next course of action is to:
    a. reassure the patient that this is a normal side effect of paclitaxel.
    b. give the patient 50mg of IV Benadryl.
    c. immediately stop the infusion and notify the oncologist.
    d. decrease the rate of paclitaxel by 50%.

3. A 62-year-old male patient diagnosed with stage 3 small cell lung cancer is admitted to the oncology unit with somnolence, weakness, nausea, vomiting, and diffuse abdominal pain. His wife reports that he has become increasingly weak over the past three days and has exhibited a change in mental status. She reports that he has not had a bowel movement in five days. Which of the following oncologic complications is a likely explanation for the patient's clinical presentation?
    a. Superior vena cava syndrome
    b. Septic shock
    c. Liver metastasis
    d. Hypercalcemia

4. Which of the following chemotherapeutic agents is classified as a Vinca alkaloid?
    a. Docetaxel
    b. Topotecan
    c. Oxaliplatin
    d. Etoposide

5. Which of the following treatment examples best describes adjuvant therapy?
    a. A 53-year-old patient receives chemotherapy and radiation for a diagnosis of stage 3 breast cancer.
    b. A 64-year-old patient diagnosed with stage 3 ovarian cancer receives chemotherapy after undergoing a total abdominal hysterectomy and bilateral salpingo-oophorectomy.
    c. A 42-year-old patient diagnosed with stage 1 breast cancer undergoes a lumpectomy with lymph node biopsy.
    d. An 80-year-old patient diagnosed with chronic leukemia receives oral chemotherapy with regular monitoring by her oncologist.

- 4 -

6. A 60-year-old male patient newly diagnosed with small cell carcinoma of the right lung is admitted to the oncology unit with a chief complaint of facial and neck swelling as well as a cough. A diagnosis of superior vena cava syndrome is made. Which of the following treatment options would you expect to see ordered for this patient?
    a. Thoracentesis under local anesthesia
    b. Chemotherapy with adjuvant radiation therapy
    c. Transfusion of two units of packed red blood cells
    d. Surgical consultation to place a chest tube

7. Which of the following would you include as part of discharge instructions for a patient diagnosed with head and neck cancer and who has received radiation therapy?
    a. Apply soothing ointments to the lips for dryness and cracking.
    b. Use a soft, nylon toothbrush when brushing teeth.
    c. Rinse the mouth several times per day with a baking soda and warm water solution.
    d. Moisten foods with sauces, gravies and other liquids.
    e. All of the above.
    f. None of the above.

8. Which chromosome is associated with chronic myelogenous leukemia?
    a. Chromosome 7
    b. Philadelphia chromosome
    c. Chromosome 13
    d. P53

9. A patient presents with a new diagnosis of non-small cell lung cancer. In the patient's medical record you learn that the tumor in the right lung is 4 cm x 6 cm and has invaded the visceral pleura. There is evidence of metastases in the mediastinal and subcarinal nodes as well as distant metastasis in the liver. Based on TNM staging, you realize that the patient has which stage of non-small cell lung cancer?
    a. Stage 2
    b. Stage 3a
    c. Stage 3b
    d. Stage 4

10. Which of the following is an example of a "B symptom" associated with lymphoma?
    a. Headache
    b. Painful lymph nodes
    c. Night sweats
    d. Edema

11. A 25-year-old female patient newly diagnosed with stage 4 Hodgkin's lymphoma presents to the outpatient oncology unit for her first dose of chemotherapy. You receive orders to administer ABVD. Which of the following would be appropriate to teach the patient regarding her chemotherapy?

    a. "The chemotherapy will be administered intravenously. If you experience any pain or burning at your IV site, notify me right away as some of the medications can cause tissue damage if they leak out of the vein into the tissue."

    b. "Your chemotherapy drugs are considered monoclonal antibodies and may cause an allergic reaction. Please let me know if you experience fever, chills, nausea, or sweating during your infusion."

    c. "The chemotherapy you are receiving can affect your fertility and may cause birth defects. It is important that you do not try to conceive a child while receiving these medications."

    d. "The chemotherapy you are receiving is not likely to cause hair loss."

    e. A and C

    f. A, B, and C

    g. All of the above

12. Which of the following agents is classified as a tyrosine kinase inhibitor?

    a. Rituximab

    b. Bortezomib

    c. Trastuzumab

    d. Sunitinib

13. One of the most common primary cancers with a high incidence of brain metastasis includes:

    a. melanoma.

    b. non-Hodgkin's lymphoma.

    c. ovarian cancer.

    d. thyroid cancer.

14. The malignancies most associated with cardiac tamponade include all of the following except:

    a. breast cancer.

    b. lymphoma.

    c. leukemia.

    d. thyroid cancer.

15. Which of the following is the preferred route for pharmacologic prophylactic treatment of nausea and vomiting?

    a. Oral

    b. Intravenous

    c. Subcutaneous

    d. Intramuscular

16. The most common presenting symptom of bladder cancer is:

    a. a urinary tract infection.

    b. bladder spasm.

    c. gross hematuria.

    d. flank pain.

17. A 60-year-old male patient recently diagnosed with stage 2 bladder cancer presents to the outpatient infusion center for his first dose of bacille Calmette-Guerin (BCG). Which of the following is **not** appropriate to teach the patient about his BCG treatment?
a. "We will collect a urine specimen prior to your procedure to ensure that you do not have any signs of infection. If an infection is present, we will need to reschedule your treatment."
b. "We will place a catheter in your bladder to instill the medication. The catheter will be clamped to keep the medication inside the bladder and we will reposition you frequently to ensure the medication is dispersed throughout the bladder."
c. "Burning, frequency, and urgency are abnormal side effects. You should notify your physician right away if any of these side effects occur."
d. "After we remove the catheter from your bladder, we will have you urinate to ensure that you are able to void and to dispose of contaminated urine."

18. The standard treatment for a bladder tumor that invades surrounding muscle is:
a. chemotherapy.
b. radiation therapy.
c. surgical intervention by radical cystectomy.
d. laser treatment.

19. Which of the following conditions are **not** associated with renal cell carcinomas?
a. Hypertension
b. Cushing's syndrome
c. Non-metastatic hepatopathy
d. Plummer-Vinson syndrome

20. The most common metastatic sites of renal cell carcinoma include all of the following except the:
a. lung.
b. brain.
c. bone.
d. liver.

21. Which type of malignancy is most frequently diagnosed in the United States?
a. Prostate cancer
b. Breast cancer
c. Lung cancer
d. Melanoma

22. Which of the following is a risk factor for prostate cancer?
a. Increased intake of foods containing lycopene
b. Increased intake of dietary fat
c. Increased intake of dietary fiber
d. Increased number of sexual partners

23. You are working in an oncology office as a registered nurse and have a male patient who was recently diagnosed with prostate cancer. The oncologist identified a suspicious area in the prostate. The patient also has a PSA level that is markedly elevated. The patient asks you what the next steps will be. The most appropriate response would be:
    a. "We will need to make an appointment in the outpatient infusion center for your first dose of chemotherapy."
    b. "We will need to schedule a needle biopsy. This is an outpatient procedure and will give the oncologist more information to establish a diagnosis."
    c. "We will need to schedule your next follow-up appointment to see the oncologist in six months."
    d. "We will need to schedule an appointment with our research team to have you enroll in a clinical trial."

24. Which of the following is **not** a viable treatment option for a patient diagnosed with stage 4 prostate cancer?
    a. Radical prostatectomy
    b. Palliative pain management
    c. Hormonal therapy
    d. External beam radiation therapy

25. Which of the following is **not** true regarding prostatic intraepithelial neoplasia (PIN)?
    a. PIN can be characterized as high or low grade
    b. PIN is considered a premalignant lesion
    c. Low-grade PIN is correlated with a lower incidence of a subsequent carcinoma of the prostate
    d. Diagnosis of PIN is indicative of a clinically palpable tumor confined to the prostate

26. Which of the following is a clinical sign of neoplastic cardiac tamponade?
    a. Bradycardia
    b. Vasodilation
    c. Increased central venous pressure
    d. Hypertension

27. Which of the following instructions would you give to a 60-year-old male patient who recently began external beam radiation therapy for stage 3 prostate cancer?
    a. "Radiation therapy will have no effect on erectile function."
    b. "You should follow a low-residue diet and drink plenty of fluids throughout the course of your therapy."
    c. "You should not take a bath or use any topical steroids if you develop rectal irritation."
    d. "There are certain side effects related to external beam radiation therapy, but fatigue is not one of them."

28. Which of the following is an example of a taxane derivative indicated for the treatment of hormone-refractory metastatic prostate cancer in patients previously treated with a docetaxel-containing regimen?
    a. Cabazitaxel
    b. Paclitaxel
    c. Sipuleucel-T
    d. Leuprolide acetate

29. Which of the following is an example of a non-modifiable risk factor in the development of testicular cancer?
    a. Testicular trauma
    b. Viral infection
    c. Cryptorchidism
    d. Exposure to DES before birth

30. All of the following are clinical features of testicular cancer except:
    a. abdominal aching.
    b. low back pain.
    c. gynecomastia.
    d. hematuria.

31. Which of the following chemotherapeutic agents may have a side effect of dose-limiting diarrhea either early (within 24 hours of administration) or late (over 24 hours after administration)?
    a. Paclitaxel
    b. Methotrexate
    c. Irinotecan
    d. Cisplatin

32. You are a registered nurse who has just begun working in an outpatient infusion center. You have learned that the required personal protective equipment that should be worn when administering chemotherapy is:
    a. a disposable long sleeved gown, disposable nitrile or neoprene non-powdered gloves, and a plastic face shield when splashes, sprays or aerosols may occur.
    b. disposable gloves only.
    c. a disposable long-sleeved gown, N95 respirator mask, and disposable nitrile or neoprene gloves.
    d. a reusable gown and disposable nitrile or neoprene gloves.

33. Which of the following interventions are **not** recommended to minimize exposure to hazardous drugs during administration?
    a. Double gloving for administration of hazardous drugs.
    b. Inspecting gloves for visible defects prior to use.
    c. Changing gloves after each use, tear, puncture, or contamination, or after 30 minutes of use.
    d. Spiking and priming the bag in a utility room over a sink.

34. Which of the following are risk factors for malignant melanoma?
    a. Blond or red hair and marked freckling on the upper back
    b. A prior human papillomavirus infection
    c. A history of excessive alcohol intake
    d. Obesity, diabetes, and hypertension

35. You are taking care of a patient who has been recently diagnosed with non-Hodgkin's lymphoma and who is receiving his first cycle of chemotherapy. You read in the patient's medical record that he has a large tumor burden and a significantly elevated LDH level. About one hour post-chemotherapy, your patient begins vomiting and is becoming somewhat lethargic. You notice elevated T-waves on the patient's telemetry. You review the patient's lab work post- chemotherapy and find the following values: sodium: 135, potassium: 6.8, calcium 7.5, and phosphorus 5.0. Which of the following is the most likely cause of this patient's symptoms?
- a. Syndrome of inappropriate antidiuretic hormone secretion (SIADH)
- b. Tumor lysis syndrome
- c. An anaphylactic reaction to chemotherapy
- d. Septic shock

36. You are caring for a patient with acute leukemia who has now developed disseminated intravascular coagulation (DIC). In DIC, the platelet count is:
- a. increased.
- b. unaffected.
- c. decreased.
- d. dependent on the fibrinogen level.

37. You are caring for a patient diagnosed with breast cancer who received chemotherapy ten days ago. At the start of your shift, you assess the patient and find the following:
    T 102.5, HR 142, BP 80/40, RR 32 breaths/minute
The patient's husband states that she has had "shaking chills" for approximately 30 minutes and has become increasingly lethargic over the past two hours. The nurse on the prior shift administered two 500 ml Normal Saline fluid boluses per physician orders for the patient's hypotension. The patient's blood pressure is 80/40 mmHg after the fluid boluses. You suspect the patient may be experiencing which of the following?
- a. Tumor lysis syndrome
- b. Anaphylaxis
- c. Septic shock
- d. Hypercalcemia

38. Which of the following interventions is **not** appropriate for teaching a patient about the prevention of lymphedema?
- a. Never allow an injection or a blood draw in the affected extremity.
- b. Do not wear tight jewelry or elastic bands around the affected extremity.
- c. Ensure that nails are manicured regularly, including cutting the cuticles.
- d. Use an electric razor to remove hair from under the arms and on the lower extremities.

39. The presence of epidermal growth factor receptor (EGFR) has been associated with which of the following?
- a. Less-aggressive tumors
- b. A worse prognosis
- c. Receptiveness to endocrine therapy
- d. Decreased rate of cancer recurrence

40. Which of the following agents is an example of an EGFR inhibitor?
   a. Bevacizumab
   b. Imatinib
   c. Lapatinib
   d. Gemtuzumab

41. An example of an unconjugated MAb approved for therapeutic use in oncology is:
   a. trastuzumab.
   b. gemtuzumab.
   a. ibritumomab.
   b. iodine-131 tositumomab.

42. All of the following are examples of anticancer agents that might be attached to conjugated MAbs except:
   a. radioactive isotopes.
   b. chemotherapeutic agents.
   c. toxins.
   d. hormones.

43. A conjugated MAb with a radioactive isotope component used in combination with rituximab for the treatment of B-cell lymphoma is:
   a. gemtuzumab.
   b. ibritumomab.
   c. iodine-131 tositumomab.
   d. alemtuzumab.

44. All of the following are true regarding estrogen receptor (ER) positive tumors except:
   a. they are well differentiated.
   b. they tend to have a prolonged overall survival compared to ER-negative tumors.
   c. they are more likely to respond to and benefit from endocrine therapy.
   d. they are more likely to respond to and benefit from chemotherapy.

45. The leading cause of cancer deaths among women is from:
   a. breast cancer.
   b. lung cancer.
   c. melanoma.
   d. ovarian cancer.

46. All of the following are potential physiologic causes for anxiety in patients diagnosed with advanced cancer except:
   a. hormone-secreting tumors.
   b. hypoxia.
   c. poorly-controlled pain.
   d. hypercalcemia.

47. You are caring for a patient with advanced lung cancer who has been experiencing bouts of anxiety throughout the course of his hospitalization. All of the following statements regarding anxiety are true except:

a. Serious anxiety reactions occur in approximately 35% of patients with advanced cancer.

b. Physical signs and symptoms of anxiety may include tachycardia, tachypnea and hypertension.

c. Prior to initiating pharmacologic intervention, the nurse should teach the patient relaxation techniques to cope with his anxiety.

d. If the patient is experiencing pain, ensure that the pain is controlled before properly evaluating anxiety.

48. All of the following medications are useful in the treatment of anxiety except:

a. lorazepam 0.5-2mg every 3-6 hours.

b. haloperidol 0.5-1.5mg every 4-6 hours.

c. midazolam 2-10mg SQ or IM once daily.

d. dicyclomine 20mg every 6 hours.

49. Which of the following statements is true regarding the pharmacologic treatment of insomnia in cancer patients?

a. Administer the highest dose of the hypnotic medication and then reduce the dose by 30-50% as insomnia resolves.

b. Do not abruptly discontinue hypnotic drugs. Instead, taper the doses over several days.

c. Instruct the patient to use the hypnotic medication every night until his symptoms resolve.

d. Hypnotic medications need to be prescribed for at least 4-6 weeks before the patient will begin to see their effectiveness.

50. Which of the following are the most common sources of bone metastases?

a. Breast, prostate and lung cancers

b. Prostate, colon and ovarian cancers

c. Lung, renal and thyroid cancers

d. Breast, lung and colon cancers

51. The most painful site of metastasis in breast or prostate cancer is the:

a. liver.

b. lungs.

c. femur.

d. brain.

52. Osteolytic bone lesions are most commonly associated with which type of cancer?

a. Gastrointestinal cancer

b. Multiple myeloma

c. Thyroid cancer

d. Prostate cancer

53. The treatment of choice for the pain associated with **localized** bone metastases is:
    a. Cox-2 inhibitors.
    b. chemotherapy.
    c. external beam radiation therapy.
    d. kyphoplasty.

54. Which of the following statements is true regarding the use of bisphosphonates in the management of bone metastases?
    a. Bisphosphonates can only be given intravenously.
    b. Bisphosphonates are only effective in alleviating bone pain associated with osteoblastic types of lesions.
    c. Bisphosphonates should be given as a preventive measure to patients with bone metastases from breast cancer or multiple myeloma.
    d. Bisphosphonates are indicated in the treatment of hypocalcemia.

55. Which of the following tumors are rarely or never associated with hypercalcemia?
    a. Breast cancer
    b. Multiple myeloma
    c. Thyroid cancer
    d. Prostate cancer

56. You are taking care of a 45-year-old patient who was recently diagnosed with acute myeloid leukemia. She has been febrile for the last two nights with a temperature of 100.5. Several diagnostic tests have been performed to rule out infection. The resident physician on duty tells you the patient has "a fever of unknown origin." The most likely cause for the patient's febrile state is:
    a. a febrile drug reaction.
    b. neutropenia.
    c. neoplastic fever.
    d. a side effect of chemotherapy.

57. Which of the following statements is true regarding pruritus in cancer patients?
    a. The incidence and severity of pruritus are related to the bilirubin level in patients with obstructive hepatobiliary disease.
    b. Pruritus is a B symptom that is often present in Hodgkin's disease.
    c. Pruritus is often associated with hypothyroidism in cancer patients.
    d. Pruritus occurs in approximately 25% of dialysis patients.

58. You are caring for a 63-year-old female patient who has been diagnosed with stage 3 pancreatic cancer. Approximately four months ago, she underwent an endoscopic retrograde cholangiopancreatography (ERCP) and was diagnosed with obstructive jaundice. The patient had a biliary stent placed to alleviate the obstruction. You are performing a clinical assessment and find that the patient is febrile with an oral temperature of 102.5. She is experiencing shaking chills and is diaphoretic. She complains of severe abdominal pain and pruritus, her urine is dark tea colored, and she appears jaundiced. The most likely cause of this patient's symptoms is:
    a. liver metastasis.
    b. a small bowel obstruction.
    c. a failure of the biliary stent.
    d. sepsis.

59. Persistent or intractable hiccups in terminally ill patients are most likely to be caused by all of the following except:
  a. irritation of the vagus nerve due to tumors of the neck, lung, or mediastinum.
  b. pharmacologic agents such as IV corticosteroids, barbiturates, or benzodiazepines.
  c. gastric distension caused by impaired gastric motility.
  d. hyponatremia related to polydipsia.

60. Which of the following statements is true regarding nausea and vomiting in cancer patients?
  a. Nausea and vomiting occur in up to 60% of patients receiving opioids, especially at the initiation of treatment.
  b. Nausea and vomiting are rare in a terminal patient's last week of life.
  c. Nausea and vomiting are particularly prevalent in patients with leukemias and lymphomas.
  d. Drug therapy for nausea and vomiting is less effective if given prophylactically.

61. After a certain dose has been given of non-opioid analgesics, further increases in dosage will not provide more analgesia. This is called a(n) ___ effect.
  a. synergistic
  b. ceiling
  c. analgesic
  d. antagonistic

62. _____ pain is the type of pain usually associated with damage to bones, soft tissues, or internal organs.
  a. Neuropathic
  b. Breakthrough
  c. Nociceptive
  d. Idiopathic

63. An example of a nociceptive pain syndrome might be:
  a. diabetic neuropathy.
  b. bone metastases.
  c. fibromyalgia.
  d. complex regional pain syndrome.

64. The principle of double effect is defined as:
  a. the difference between providing analgesic medications that might inadvertently hasten death versus providing medication to intentionally cause death.
  b. the difference between developing a state of tolerance to a medication versus forming a psychological dependence on a medication.
  c. an outcome occurring between two or more medications that produce effects that are greater than the sum of the two.
  d. tolerance to a drug that develops through continued use of another drug with similar pharmacologic actions.

65. The World Health Organization (WHO) has summarized the principles of pain management in cancer patients by all of the following methods **except** by:
   a. mouth.
   b. the clock.
   c. analgesic ladder.
   d. the diagnosis.

66. Which of the following medications may be useful in the treatment of neuropathic pain?
   a. Codeine 60 mg q 4 hours with an NSAID
   b. Dexamethasone 16 mg daily
   c. An opioid plus carbamazepine 200 mg twice daily
   d. Diazepam 10 mg at bedtime q hs

67. You are taking care of a patient with advanced cancer who is having a significant amount of pain. Which of the following statements from the patient indicate that he has an understanding of his morphine prescription?
   a. "I am hesitant to take my morphine because I am afraid I will stop breathing."
   b. "I prefer not to take narcotics. I do not have much time left and I feel that if I take narcotics it will hasten my death."
   c. "Morphine makes me nauseated, so I know I am allergic to it."
   d. "I know that I need more morphine because my disease has progressed, not because I have a psychological dependence."

68. Which of the following statements is true regarding how opioids affect gastrointestinal function?
   a. Opioids cause decreased muscle tone in the gastric antrum, the small intestine, and the colon.
   b. Opioids decrease segmental contractions of the bowel.
   c. Opioids increase stool frequency and volume.
   d. Opioids increase water and electrolyte absorption from the gut lumen.

69. Ascites occurs most commonly in patients with which type of primary malignancy?
   a. Ovarian cancer
   b. Colon cancer
   c. Pancreatic cancer
   d. Endometrial cancer

70. Which of the following statements is true related to ascites in the cancer patient?
   a. Ascites primarily affects patients with liver cancer because of tumor invasion in the liver parenchyma.
   b. Bulging flanks may become apparent in a clinical assessment when there is more than 250 ml of fluid in the abdomen.
   c. Peritoneal carcinomatosis is the most common cause of ascites in cancer patients.
   d. Patients with ascites rarely respond to diuretics and often require paracentesis.

71. Which of the following statements is true regarding brain metastases?
    a. Brain metastases occur in 25-35% of all cancer patients.
    b. Brain metastases most commonly occur in patients with a primary gastrointestinal cancer diagnosis.
    c. Brain metastases are less common than primary brain tumors.
    d. Brain metastases are more likely to be multiple as opposed to solitary.

72. The most common presenting symptom in brain metastasis is:
    a. a seizure.
    b. ataxia.
    c. focal weakness.
    d. a headache.

73. Excluding brain metastasis, which of the following may cause seizures in patients with advanced cancer?
    a. Hyponatremia
    b. Hypoxemia
    c. Sepsis
    d. All of the above

74. Which of the following statements is true regarding the Karnofsky Performance Scale?
    a. The higher the Karnofsky score, the worse prognosis for most serious illnesses.
    b. The Karnofsky Performance Scale allows patients to be classified according to their functional impairment.
    c. The Karnofsky Performance Scale is ineffective when comparing different therapies and assessing the prognosis of individual patients.
    d. All of the above

75. Which of the following symptoms is the most accurate marker of depression in a patient with advanced cancer?
    a. Weight loss
    b. Diminished concentration
    c. Feelings of worthlessness
    d. Insomnia

76. Which of the following factors should be considered when performing a sexual health assessment?
    a. Obtain the sexual health assessment after you have had time to get to know the patient.
    b. Begin with more sensitive topics and move to less sensitive topics throughout the assessment.
    c. Include the patient's goals for treatment in your assessment.
    d. All of the above

77. The PLISSIT model is frequently used for sexuality assessments and counseling. The "P" in PLISSIT stands for:
    a. permission.
    b. plan of care.
    c. preparation.
    d. potential concerns.

78. You are caring for a patient recently diagnosed with advanced cancer who is struggling to find meaning in his diagnosis. He states, "I just don't understand why this is happening to me." Which of the following is a suitable response to facilitate discussion around the meaning of his illness?

    a. "A lot of people are diagnosed with cancer so it is not only you experiencing these types of feelings."

    b. "How often do you talk with your family about your illness and how it has impacted your lives?"

    c. "Have you ever known anyone with advanced cancer? How did they cope?"

    d. "You are probably feeling this way because you have never struggled with an illness before."

79. All of the following are types of allogeneic bone marrow transplants except:

    a. syngeneic.

    b. related.

    c. autologous.

    d. unrelated.

80. Which of the following tests would **not** be included in a routine pre-transplant evaluation for a patient preparing to receive a bone marrow transplant?

    a. Dental consult

    b. Hepatitis screen

    c. PET scan

    d. ABO and Rh typing

81. Which of the following statements is true regarding radiation pneumonitis?

    a. It occurs immediately following radiation therapy.

    b. It is treated with steroids.

    c. It occurs frequently in patients receiving radiation; however, it is not dose limiting.

    d. It is not dose dependent.

82. The process by which normal cells are transformed into cancer cells is known as:

    a. metastasis.

    b. carcinomatosis.

    c. carcinogenesis.

    d. meiosis.

83. Which of the following statements regarding the Medicare Hospice benefit is false?

    a. Individual patients must be entitled to Part A of Medicare and be certified as terminally ill in order to be eligible to elect hospice care.

    b. The medical prognosis of the patient electing hospice care is defined as a life expectancy of six months or less.

    c. An individual patient or his authorized representative must elect hospice care in order to receive it.

    d. A registered nurse or hospice case manager must certify the patient as being terminally ill in order to be eligible to elect hospice care.

84. Which of the following statements is true regarding palliative sedation therapy?
    a. It is also referred to as passive euthanasia.
    b. It can be initiated in the home setting as long as the patient is under hospice care.
    c. It's goal is symptom management and not hastening death.
    d. It should be initiated prior to imminent death.

85. Cell-cycle specific drugs include which of the following classes of chemotherapeutic agents?
    a. Anti-metabolites
    b. Antitumor antibiotics
    c. Alkylating agents
    d. Nitrosoureas

86. Which of the following chemotherapeutic agents has the highest emetogenic potential?
    a. Paclitaxel
    b. Carboplatin
    c. Cytarabine
    d. Cisplatin

87. You are caring for a patient who recently received chemotherapy for a diagnosis of lung cancer. Your patient expresses an interest in acupuncture and asks if you can provide him with more information on the benefits. Which of the following responses illustrates your understanding of using acupuncture among cancer patients?
    a. "Acupuncture is likely to cause an infection and should not be done until you are in remission."
    b. "There is no data to support that acupuncture will improve your symptoms."
    c. "There has been research that supports acupuncture to be very effective in relieving the nausea and vomiting caused by chemotherapy treatment."
    d. "I don't believe in alternative therapies. I only support conventional treatment options."

88. During which phase of a clinical trial for a new anti-cancer drug is the overall benefit versus the risk of the drug evaluated and more information regarding safety and efficacy established?
    a. Phase 1
    b. Phase 2
    c. Phase 3
    d. Phase 4

89. Which of the following is **not** a kinetic characteristic of cancer cells?
    a. Inability to differentiate
    b. Chromosomal instability
    c. Capacity to metastasize
    d. Controlled proliferation

90. The most frequently diagnosed malignancy in HIV-infected patients is:
    a. Kaposi's sarcoma.
    b. B-cell lymphoma.
    c. acute myelogenous leukemia.
    d. multiple myeloma.

91. The most common symptom of cancer is:
    a. nausea and vomiting.
    b. pain.
    c. fatigue.
    d. mucositis.

92. You are caring for a patient who was recently diagnosed with breast cancer and who is receiving hormonal therapy. Which of the following would you include when teaching the patient about the side effects of hormonal therapy?
    a. "The hormonal agent you are taking should not affect your sexuality."
    b. "The hormonal agent you are taking can cause adverse fetal effects, including loss. You should avoid becoming pregnant during treatment and for at least two months after your treatment is discontinued."
    c. "Certain hormonal agents can decrease the risk of pregnancy."
    d. "Hormonal agents are unlikely to cause disruptions to your menstrual cycle."

93. A patient is admitted to the oncology unit with a new diagnosis of colon cancer. The patient undergoes a surgical resection and is ready to be discharged. His physician says that he will be starting chemotherapy next month and will receive 5-fluorouracil along with bevacizumab. The patient expresses concern over having to wait so long to start his chemotherapy. Which of the following statements is the best response to explain the reason for the delay?
    a. "The chemotherapy you are going to receive can cause complications in wound healing. It is inadvisable to initiate this type of chemotherapy for at least 28 days following major surgery."
    b. "The chemotherapy you are going to receive can cause hypotension. We need to wait until your condition is more stable to begin chemotherapy."
    c. "All of our patients must wait at least thirty days after surgery to begin chemotherapy."
    d. "Next month is the soonest the infusion center can schedule your chemotherapy."

94. Which of the following statements is true regarding survivorship?
    a. Cancer survival begins when the patient is in remission.
    b. There are four phases of cancer survivorship: denial, anger, depression, and acceptance.
    c. Survivorship focuses on physiologic effects including the long-term effects of treatment.
    d. Survivorship issues also affect the support system of the survivor including family, friends and co-workers.

95. You are caring for a patient who recently lost his wife to cancer. He has been admitted for chest pain and shortness of breath. In talking with the patient's children, they share with you that their father has been acting as if nothing has happened and is coping surprisingly well. You suspect the patient may be experiencing which type of grief?
    a. Chronic
    b. Conflicted
    c. Absent or Delayed
    d. Normal

96. Ipilimumab is a monoclonal antibody approved for the treatment of unresectable or metastatic melanoma. Ipilimumab can cause severe and fatal immune-mediated adverse reactions most commonly manifested as which of the following?
    a. Enterocolitis
    b. Hypertension
    c. Vasculitis
    d. Autoimmune thyroiditis

97. Which of the following proteasome inhibitors is indicated for the treatment of relapsed or refractory multiple myeloma?
    a. Thalidomide
    b. Omalizumab
    c. Lapatinib
    d. Carfilzomib

98. Which of the following statements is true regarding chemotherapy-induced peripheral neuropathy (CIPN)?
    a. Lower extremity symptoms such as numbness, tingling, weakness, and loss of proprioception affect the fine motor skills of the patient.
    b. Patients experiencing CIPN should be told to rest as much as possible and to minimize physical activity.
    c. Pharmacologic management of neuropathic pain is limited to anticonvulsants such as gabapentin and pregabalin.
    d. Patients receiving chemotherapy should be assessed at every visit for symptoms such as numbness, tingling, or discomfort in the upper or lower extremities.

99. You are caring for a 49-year-old female patient who was diagnosed with breast cancer two years ago. She is currently taking tamoxifen. The patient shares with you that her physician recently started her on bupropion for depression. Which of the following is true regarding the patient's treatment with tamoxifen?
    a. Tamoxifen often causes depression in patients.
    b. Bupropion is a strong inhibitor of CYP2D6, the primary mediator that converts tamoxifen to its active metabolites. Bupropion should not be used concomitantly with tamoxifen.
    c. Bupropion is not an inhibitor of CYP2D6 and can be used in the treatment of depression for patients receiving tamoxifen.
    d. Patients taking tamoxifen should avoid all antidepressant medications.

100. The clinical manifestations of multiple myeloma can by summarized by the acronym CRAB. What does the A in CRAB stand for?
    a. Abdominal pain
    b. Adrenal insufficiency
    c. Anemia
    d. Anorexia

101. An example of a psychologic effect that may occur after a patient completes his cancer treatment is:
    a. peripheral neuropathy.
    b. ambivalence regarding health care follow up.
    c. employment-related problems including fear of loss of employment.
    d. an increased passion or zest for life.

102. Which of the following statements is true regarding the development of secondary cancers in cancer survivors?
    a. Secondary cancer is not likely to be caused by the treatment of the original cancer (i.e. chemotherapy or radiation therapy).
    b. Patients who received a bone marrow transplant are not at risk of developing a secondary malignancy.
    c. Cancer survivors have a 14% higher risk of developing a new cancer.
    d. There are no modifiable risk factors in the development of a secondary cancer.

103. You are caring for a 35-year-old female patient who completed treatment for Hodgkin's disease two years ago. Which of the following statements by the patient warrants further follow up by the nurse?
    a. "I have had trouble becoming pregnant since I had my cancer."
    b. "I always get my flu shot every year."
    c. "I often get sick but I make sure that I get to my doctor right away when I think I might have an infection."
    d. "I have been experiencing shortness of breath over the past month when going up and down my stairs at home."

104. Pertuzumab is a monoclonal antibody used in combination with which two chemotherapeutic agents to treat metastatic breast cancer with HER-2 expression?
    a. Cisplatin and paclitaxel
    b. Trastuzumab and docetaxel
    c. Lapatinib and trastuzumab
    d. Docetaxel and cisplatin

105. Mr. Smith is a 55-year-old patient currently undergoing treatment for prostate cancer. He is taking Vicodin as needed for pain and reports that he takes one Vicodin every six hours for pain control. He presents today complaining of abdominal fullness, bloating, and cramping and states his last bowel movement was five days ago. Mr. Smith reports that he has been regularly taking laxatives to help with his constipation but his symptoms have persisted. According to the NCI grading scale, Mr. Smith's constipation would be graded as:
    a. Grade 1
    b. Grade 2
    c. Grade 3
    d. Grade 4

106. Mrs. Jones is a 63-year-old patient with breast cancer. She is being treated with docetaxel, doxorubicin and cyclophosphamide. Mrs. Jones presents today with numbness and tingling of her fingers and toes. She reports a worsening of these symptoms over the past two months. She was unable to button her blouse or tie her shoes today due to the numbness in her fingers. She can no longer drive due to the worsening numbness in her feet. Mrs. Jones' peripheral neuropathy would be classified per the NCI grading scale as:
    a. Grade 1
    b. Grade 2
    c. Grade 3
    d. Grade 4

107. Most toxicity-grading criteria scales range from:
    a. 0-2
    b. 0-4
    c. 1-10
    d. 1-100

108. You are caring for a patient who has elected to stop treatment for his advanced metastatic cancer. He has expressed that he "just wants to be comfortable" and a do-not-resuscitate order has been written based on his wishes. His family expresses concerns while you are discontinuing the patient's intravenous fluids. Which of the following statements is most appropriate in teaching the patient's family about hydration and the end of life?
    a. "If you would like me to turn the fluids back on I will do that."
    b. "The physician wrote the order to discontinue the fluids. If you would like to speak to the physician, I will page him for you."
    c. "Lessening the amount of fluid through the IV can actually help to decrease certain symptoms such as excess congestion.
    d. "We typically do not administer fluids to patients with a do-not-resuscitate order."

109. Mr. Jones is a 50-year-old patient admitted to the oncology unit with complaints of nausea, abdominal pain, fever and fatigue. He states that he has noticed his urine has appeared much darker over the past two days. He was treated for lung cancer one year ago with chemotherapy. Additionally, Mr. Jones states he has noticed "purple splotches" on his lower extremities. His CBC shows a hemoglobin level of 8 g/dL and a platelet count of 30,000/mm3. Which of the following do you suspect Mr. Jones may be experiencing?
    a. Gastrointestinal bleed
    b. Thrombotic thrombocytopenia purpura (TTP)
    c. Von Willebrand disease
    d. Disseminated intravascular coagulation (DIC)

110. Thrombocytopenia describes:
    a. a decrease in the circulating platelets below 100,000/mm3.
    b. a decrease in the circulating white blood cells below 1500/mm3.
    c. a decrease in the circulating neutrophils below 1000/mm3.
    d. a decrease in the circulating red blood cells below 1000/mm3.

111. You are caring for a 39-year-old patient who is undergoing treatment for newly-diagnosed breast cancer. During your assessment the patient becomes tearful and states, "I just can't stand the way I look without hair. I'm sure my husband is not going to want to be with me anymore." Which of the following statements by the nurse is most appropriate to address how the patient is coping with her alteration in body image?
    a. "Don't worry, your husband will still want to be with you. Your hair will grow back."
    b. "What you are feeling is a normal response. In time you will accept it."
    c. "It is okay for you to grieve the loss of your hair and to be angry about it. Would it be okay for us to talk about some resources and options you could utilize to help with this loss?"
    d. "I would be happy to see if we can get you a turban or scarf to wear."

112. You are preparing to provide education to one of your patients prior to discharge. Which of the following should be evaluated prior to initiating the teaching?
    a. The patient's comfort level
    b. The patient's readiness to learn
    c. The patient's cognitive ability to learn
    d. All of the above

113. You are caring for a dying patient who is receiving high-dose intravenous morphine for pain management. The family reports that the patient has begun hallucinating and having "muscle twitches." What is the most likely cause of the patient's symptoms?
    a. Accumulation of opioid metabolites
    b. Dehydration
    c. Hypoxemia
    d. Ineffective pain control

114. The Patient Self-Determination Act, established in 1990, requires that all hospitals receiving federal funds must ask patients at the time of admission if:
    a. they have developmental disabilities.
    b. they have advanced directives.
    c. they wish to release any health information to a 3rd party.
    d. they would like a copy of their bill of rights.

115. You are caring for a patient who has been diagnosed with malignant melanoma and who is being treated with interferon 10 million units/m^2 SQ for 48 weeks. Which of the following clinical findings warrants further follow up by the nurse that may result in discontinuation of treatment?
    a. An oral temperature of 100 degrees
    b. A hemoglobin level of 11.5 g/dL
    c. A platelet count of 60,000/mm3
    d. A triglyceride level of 1200 mg/dL

116. Vorinostat, a targeted therapy known as a histone deacetylase inhibitor, is FDA approved for the treatment of:
    a. acute myelogenous leukemia.
    b. multiple myeloma.
    c. cutaneous T-cell lymphoma.
    d. breast cancer.

117. Which of the following statements is true regarding Totect administration for the treatment of anthracycline extravasation?
    a. Totect infusion should be initiated within two hours of extravasation.
    b. Totect is administered over the course of 48 hours.
    c. Apply ice to area of extravasation prior to Totect administration, but remove ice 15 minutes before the start of the infusion.
    d. Infusion of Totect should be initiated in the same arm as the extravasation.

118. All of the following are risk factors in the development of acute myeloid leukemia (AML) except:
    a. Down syndrome.
    b. previous chemotherapy.
    c. exposure to benzene.
    d. female gender.

119. You are caring for a patient who was diagnosed with metastatic lung cancer. The patient now has brain metastasis that was discovered after having an MRI earlier in the day. While completing your assessment, the patient begins complaining of a severe headache and nausea. The family states that he has had trouble remembering things and has exhibited some personality changes over the past two days. You notify the physician of the changes in the patient's condition. Which of the following interventions do you expect to see ordered by the physician?
    a. Lumbar puncture
    b. Stat dose of IV dexamethasone
    c. CT scan of the chest and abdomen
    d. P.o. anticonvulsant q 6 hours

120. All of the following statements are true regarding mucositis except:
    a. Mucositis can occur anywhere along the digestive tract.
    b. Mucositis is the most debilitating symptom reported by cancer patients.
    c. Patients should avoid flossing if mucositis occurs.
    d. Approximately 20-40% of patients receiving chemotherapy develop mucositis.

121. Which of the following services are not covered under the Hospice Medicare Benefit?
    a. Speech therapy
    b. Short-term inpatient care
    c. Medical equipment
    d. Room and board

122. You are caring for a patient who was recently diagnosed with advanced cancer. The patient begins asking you questions regarding his prognosis and is expressing difficulty in making decisions about advance directives. Which of the following statements is the best example of effective communication?

a. "I know that you are feeling afraid to make a decision regarding advance directives. Did your doctor tell you that nothing more can be done to treat your cancer?"

b. "Your disease has progressed so it is important for you to think about putting advance directives into place."

c. "It sounds like you are concerned about how to move forward with advance directives. Would it be ok if we discussed some of the goals you have for your care?"

d. "I will call the social worker to assist you with your decision about advance directives."

123. You are caring for a patient who is being treated with capecitabine for metastatic colorectal cancer. Which of the following statements by the patient indicates a lack of understanding of the medication?

a. "I should take this medication within a half hour after eating."

b. "I should call my doctor if I experience diarrhea that persists after I take my Imodium."

c. "I should wear sun screen and avoid sun exposure."

d. "If I miss a dose of my medication I will take it with my next scheduled dose."

124. Which of the following is true regarding the use of quadrivalent human papillomavirus recombinant vaccine (Gardasil) for the prevention of cervical cancer?

a. Gardasil is a vaccine indicated in the prevention of all gynecological malignancies.

b. Patients should be between the ages of 16 and 30 years to receive Gardasil.

c. Gardasil should be administered as an IM injection given in three separate doses.

d. A pre-treatment complete blood count and basic metabolic panel should be obtained prior to administration of Gardasil.

125. Clinical manifestations of hepatic veno-occlusive disease after a hematopoietic stem cell transplant include which of the following?

a. Hyperbilirubinemia, hepatomegaly, and jaundice

b. Jaundice, hypotension, and renal failure

c. Hepatomegaly, weight loss, and fever

d. Hypotension, fever, and right upper quadrant pain

126. Which of the following statements regarding massage therapy is an appropriate teaching point for patients considering massage as a complementary therapy?

a. Massage therapy should be avoided in cancer patients due to the risk of metastasis caused by tissue manipulation near a tumor site.

b. The American Cancer Society does not support the use of massage therapy as a complementary therapy.

c. Massage therapy can improve muscle tone and mobility and leads to increased circulation.

d. Reiki therapy is preferred over massage therapy for cancer patients.

127. Which of the following statements is true regarding genetic predisposition in cancer development?
    a. Most hereditary cancers arise from inheriting one mutated gene.
    b. There are over 20 types of inherited cancer syndromes.
    c. Familial cancers are limited to a particular type of cancer.
    d. Inherited cancers account for 20% of all cancers.

128. You are caring for a patient with small cell lung cancer who was admitted to the oncology unit for nausea, vomiting, oliguria, and confusion. The patient's wife states that he has become increasingly lethargic over the past three days. His basic metabolic panel shows the following: sodium 121 mEq/L, potassium 3.2 mEq/L, CO2 23 mmol/L, BUN 9 mg/dL, creatinine 0.4 mg/dL, and glucose 110 mg/dl. The physician makes a diagnosis of SIADH. Which of the following do you expect will be ordered for your patient?
    a. Diuresis with furosemide 0.5-1.0mg/kg
    b. Pamidronate 90 mg IV over 2 hours
    c. Restrict fluid to 500 ml per 24 hours
    d. Hydrate with 1-2 L of isotonic saline over 2 hours.

129. Which of the following is true regarding screening guidelines for the early detection of colorectal cancer?
    a. Screening should begin at age 60.
    b. A flexible sigmoidoscopy should be performed every two years.
    c. A colonoscopy is recommended every five years.
    d. A fecal occult blood test or fecal immunochemical test should be performed every year.

130. Which of the following factors have the potential to influence the grieving process?
    a. Characteristics of the deceased
    b. History of coping
    c. Level of support
    d. All of the above

131. You are caring for a patient at the end of life who is experiencing terminal agitation. Which of the following is a potential treatable cause of terminal agitation?
    a. Constipation
    b. Dyspnea
    c. Hypercalcemia
    d. All of the above

132. Which of the following characteristics are typical of the pre-active phase of the dying process?
    a. Increased sleep
    b. No interest in food or fluid
    c. Abnormal respiratory pattern
    d. Terminal congestion

133. Which of the following is **not** a recommended non-pharmacologic treatment choice for a patient experiencing dyspnea at the end of life?
    a. Speaking in a soothing, calm voice
    b. Using a fan to promote air circulation
    c. Being present as a caregiver
    d. Increasing the room temperature

134. Which of the following should be included in an education plan designed for a patient diagnosed with head and neck cancer who is about to receive radiation therapy?
    a. Dysgeusia will be temporary and should resolve in 2-4 weeks after treatment.
    b. Steroid creams or rinses can be used to moisten the lips if xerostomia occurs.
    c. Rinse the mouth with commercial-brand mouthwash daily.
    d. If xerostomia occurs, food may be moistened with gravies and sauces.

135. Which of the following is a risk factor associated with epithelial ovarian cancer?
    a. African American race
    b. Late menarche
    c. Early menopause
    d. Nulliparity

136. Which of the following is true regarding the use of pegfilgrastim?
    a. Pegfilgrastim has increased renal clearance compared with filgrastim.
    b. Pegfilgrastim should not be administered within 14 days before chemotherapy.
    c. Pegfilgrastim is administered 12 hours after chemotherapy.
    d. Pegfilgrastim is administered as a subcutaneous injection over the course of five days post-chemotherapy.

137. Which of the following statements is false regarding dietary supplements in cancer treatment?
    a. Patients should be educated to consult their physician prior to starting a dietary supplement while undergoing cancer treatment.
    b. Ginger may be helpful in managing nausea and vomiting associated with chemotherapy.
    c. A diet high in antioxidants is recommended for patients undergoing chemotherapy.
    d. Flaxseed is an herbal supplement that may enhance immune function.

138. Sodium thiosulfate is the recommended antidote for the extravasation of which class of chemotherapeutic agents?
    a. Anti-tumor antibiotics
    b. Vinca alkaloids
    c. Taxanes
    d. Alkylating agents

139. All of the following are true regarding fatigue in cancer patients except:
    a. fatigue is the most common symptom cancer patients experience.
    b. the prevalence of severe fatigue in patients with advanced cancer is approximately 75%.
    c. cancer fatigue is usually relieved by sleep or rest.
    d. fatigue often presents with pain, insomnia, and depression or anxiety.

140. Which of the following is an example of a metabolic change caused by a malignancy?
    a. Increased protein degradation
    b. Decreased rate of gluconeogenesis
    c. Hyperalbuminemia
    d. Positive nitrogen balance

141. Which of the following statistics is true regarding cancer survivors?
    a. The majority of cancer survivors are younger than age 65.
    b. Men make up the largest proportion of cancer survivors.
    c. Breast cancer survivors are the largest group of cancer survivors.
    d. The number of cancer survivors has decreased over the past decade.

142. Which of the following ethnic groups has the lowest overall cancer incidence and mortality?
    a. African American
    b. Asian/Pacific Islander
    c. Native American
    d. Hispanic

143. All of the following statements should be included when teaching a patient about how to get health information from an Internet source except:
    a. Verify when the website was posted to ensure the information is current.
    b. Verify who created the website and ensure it is from a reputable institution.
    c. Assume that most information posted on websites is screened for accuracy before it is posted.
    d. Ensure the website has sources or references posted from reputable studies.

144. Which of the following best describes systemic inflammatory response syndrome (SIRS) manifestation?
    a. Heart rate greater than 120 beats per minute and respiratory rate greater than 28 breaths per minute.
    b. Temperature greater than 38.5 degrees Celsius and more than 20% bands.
    c. White blood cell count greater than 15,000 and PaCO2 less than 32 mm Hg.
    d. Temperature greater than 38 degrees Celsius and heart rate greater than 90 beats per minute.

145. Which of the following groups of chemotherapeutic agents has the highest potential for neurotoxicity?
    a. Ifosfamide, vinblastine, vincristine
    b. Cisplatin, thiotepa, mitomycin C
    c. Cyclophosphamide, melphalan, vinblastine
    d. Paclitaxel, 5-fluorouracil, cytarabine

146. The two classes of chemotherapeutic agents that are most likely to cause arthralgias and myalgias are:
    a. Alkylating agents and anti-metabolites
    b. Anti-hormonal agents and nitrosoureas
    c. Anti-tumor antibiotics and monoclonal antibodies
    d. Vinca plant alkaloids and taxanes

147. Which of the following could be utilized as a preventive strategy in the management of cancer-related pain?
    a. Instruct the patient to only take prescribed analgesics when their pain level is moderate to severe to prevent narcotic dependency.
    b. The use of bone-modifying agents to prevent skeletal events including fractures and bone pain caused by bone metastases.
    c. Avoid the use of adjuvant agents or coanalgesics.
    d. The pharmacologic management of pain should begin with mild opioids.

148. An example of an antibody-drug conjugate (ADC) monoclonal antibody is:
    a. Ibritumomab tiuxetan (Zevalin)
    b. Ado-trastuzumab emtansine (Kadcyla or TDM-1)
    c. Alemtuzumab (Campath)
    d. Cetuximab (Erbitux)

149. You are caring for a patient with chronic lymphocytic leukemia (CLL) who arrives at the outpatient infusion center for her first dose of ofatumumab. Approximately 30 minutes into the infusion, the patient begins to complain of nausea, flushing, and chills. You check the patient's vital signs and note the patient's blood pressure to be 80/42. Which type of infusion reaction best describes the reaction the patient is experiencing?
    a. Cytokine-release reaction
    b. Cytotoxic
    c. IgE-mediated
    d. Adverse drug reaction

150. You are caring for a patient who experienced an infusion reaction during her first dose of ofatumumab. The patient experienced nausea, flushing, chills, and hypotension. You initiated a rapid response team. Initially, the patient appeared to be doing better with the administration of antihistamines and IV fluids; however, the patient is now experiencing a recurrence of symptoms, including shortness of breath and hypotension. The patient is going to be admitted to the intensive care unit. Which of the following classifications according to the National Cancer Institute Common Terminology Criteria for Adverse Events (CTCAE) for cytokine-release syndrome best describes the patient's presentation?
    a. Grade I
    b. Grade II
    c. Grade III
    d. Grade IV
    e. Grade V

151. Which of the following is true regarding cancer survivorship?
    a. A cancer survivor is defined as anyone who has received cancer treatment and is considered to be in remission.
    b. Approximately one-third of people diagnosed with cancer are expected to live 5 years or more after diagnosis.
    c. In 2006, the Institute of Medicine (IOM) recommended that cancer survivors receive an individualized survivorship care plan.
    d. Survivorship begins at the end of treatment and continues until recurrence.

152. Certain viruses and bacteria have been linked in the development of various cancers. Which of the following is not a true statement regarding the link between viral infection and cancer development?
    a. Helicobacter pylori has been shown to increase the risk of gastric cancer.
    b. Hepatitis B and C increase the risk for liver cancer.
    c. Human papillomavirus (HPV) increases the risk for cervical cancer.
    d. Cytomegalovirus increases the risk of renal cell carcinoma.

153. Which of the following malignancies carries a high probability for hemorrhage?
    a. acute promyelocytic leukemia (APL)
    b. chronic lymphocytic leukemia (CLL)
    c. glioblastoma
    d. choriocarcinoma

154. You are caring for a patient with mantle cell lymphoma who is receiving Ibrutinib (Imbruvica). When teaching the patient about common adverse effects of the medication, you include all of the following except:
    a. thrombocytopenia
    b. diarrhea
    c. hypokalemia
    d. musculoskeletal pain

155. According to the National Comprehensive Cancer Network (NCCN), febrile neutropenia is defined as:
    a. an absolute neutrophil count of less than 500 cells/mm3 or an absolute neutrophil count of 1,000 cells/mm3 predicted to decline to less than 500 cells/mm3 over the next 48 hours.
    b. an absolute neutrophil count of less than 1,500 cells/mm3
    c. an absolute neutrophil count of less than 1,000 cells/mm3
    d. an absolute neutrophil count of less than 200 cells/mm3 or an absolute neutrophil count of 500 cells/mm3 predicted to decline to less than 200 cells/mm3 over the next 24 hours.

156. Which of the following is true regarding screening for cervical cancer?
    a. Screening should begin at age 16, regardless of the age of onset of sexual activity.
    b. Women who have received the HPV vaccination should be screened less frequently than women who have not received the vaccination.
    c. Screening should be performed annually.
    d. Screening for women 21-29 years of age is recommended every 3 years.

157. You working in an outpatient clinic and about to provide a patient with education on colon cancer screening. Which of the following statements by the patient indicates a need for further education regarding colon cancer screening recommendations?
    a. "I should begin getting screened at age 50."
    b. "My physician may order a colonoscopy or a test that detects blood in my stool as part of the screening process."
    c. "Since my brother has colorectal polyps, my physician may want to screen me sooner than age 50."
    d. "I will have a colonoscopy every 3 years as part of my screening for colon cancer."

158. Ramucirumab (Cyramza) is a recombinant monoclonal antibody that was approved by the FDA in 2014 for the treatment of:
    a. advanced or metastatic gastric or gastroesophageal junction adenocarcinoma.
    b. advanced or metastatic renal cell carcinoma
    c. previously treated advanced or metastatic lung cancer
    d. previously untreated chronic lymphocytic leukemia

159. You are working with a new registered nurse on the oncology unit. Her patient is receiving fluorouracil and she is preparing to educate her on oral hygiene care. Which of the following teaching points should she include in her teaching?
    a. Avoid toothpastes containing fluoride
    b. Use an electric toothbrush 3-4 times daily
    c. Use a toothpaste with a neutral taste that contains fluoride
    d. Avoid flossing

160. Which of the following interventions could be utilized in the management of xerostomia?
    a. Instruct the patient to choose soft foods to minimize chewing.
    b. Encourage the patient to chew gum or consume hard candy.
    c. Consider the use of a sialogogue to increase salivary flow.
    d. Avoid toothpastes or oral care products containing fluoride.

161. Pembrolizumab (Keytruda) is a monoclonal antibody recently approved for the treatment of advanced melanoma. Pembrolizumab is a:
    a. recombinant, chimeric monoclonal antibody directed against the epidermal growth factor (EGFR).
    b. recombinant, DNA-derived humanized monoclonal antibody directed against the cell surface glycoprotein CD52.
    c. humanized monoclonal IgG4 antibody directed against human cell surface receptor PD-1 (programmed cell death).
    d. recombinant humanized monoclonal antibody directed against the human epidermal growth factor receptor 2 (HER-2).

162. Aprepitant is an antiemetic agent used in the treatment of chemotherapy-induced nausea and vomiting (CINV). Aprepitant is classified as a:
    a. 5HT3 receptor antagonist
    b. NK1 receptor antagonist
    c. dopamine receptor antagonist
    d. corticosteroid

163. You are caring for a patient in the outpatient infusion center who has been receiving irinotecan. During your assessment of the patient, he states that he has been experiencing an increase in liquid stools. He had been having approximately 3 bowel movements per day and now he has been having upwards of 7-9 diarrhea stools per day. According the National Cancer Institute's Common Terminology Criteria for Adverse Events (CTCAE), the patient's diarrhea would be graded as a:
    a. Grade 1
    b. Grade 2
    c. Grade 3
    d. Grade 4

164. Sensory symptoms of chemotherapy-induced peripheral neuropathy may include all of the following except:
    a. pain
    b. loss of sensation
    c. difficulty distinguishing hot and cold
    d. ringing in the ears

165. Which of the following chemotherapeutic agents is not likely to cause chemotherapy-induced peripheral neuropathy?
    a. Vincristine
    b. Cisplatin
    c. Bortezomib
    d. 5-Fluorouracil

Answers and Explanations

1. C: A bone marrow biopsy is not routinely performed as part of a diagnostic work-up for colorectal cancer. Barium enemas provide a clear picture of the large intestine and are useful in detection of smaller tumors. Colonoscopy provides increased visualization and the ability to biopsy lesions. CEA is elevated in later stages of colorectal cancer and may have prognostic value at diagnosis or disease recurrence.

2. C: The patient is experiencing signs of an infusion reaction with the potential for anaphylaxis. The nurse must be alert to recognize signs and symptoms of an early infusion reaction to avoid an anaphylactic response. The first step in addressing an infusion reaction is to immediately stop the infusion and notify the physician.

3. D: Hypercalcemia is the oncologic complication that presents with symptoms of mental status change, weakness, nausea, vomiting, constipation, and abdominal pain. Small cell lung cancer is a malignancy commonly associated with hypercalcemia. Superior vena cava syndrome presents as edema of the face, neck, and upper extremities; respiratory compromise, chest pain, headache, dizziness and a feeling of facial fullness. The clinical features of septic shock include tachypnea, nausea, diarrhea, confusion, and ultimately oliguria and metabolic acidosis. The patient may experience some of these same symptoms with liver metastasis as well.

4. D: Vinca alkaloids are a class of chemotherapeutic agents that exert their cytotoxic effects by binding to microtubular proteins during the metaphase of the cell cycle, causing mitotic arrest. Etoposide is a Vinca alkaloid. Docetaxel is a taxane derivative. Topotecan is a topoisomerase I inhibitor. Oxaliplatin is an anti-metabolite.

5. B: Adjuvant therapy is an additional cancer treatment given after the primary treatment to minimize the risk of cancer recurrence. In example b, the patient underwent surgery as a primary treatment with chemotherapy given as adjuvant therapy. Primary treatment is defined as the first treatment given and is also referred to as first line treatment, induction treatment, or primary therapy.

6. B: The correct answer is chemotherapy with adjuvant radiation therapy to shrink the tumor and to elevate the obstruction that is causing the syndrome. Thoracentesis and chest tube placement would be viable treatment options for a pleural effusion. Transfusion of packed red blood cells would not be a suitable treatment option for superior vena cava syndrome.

7. E: Patients diagnosed with head and neck cancer who are being treated with radiation therapy are at risk for oral mucositis. Application of soothing ointments for dryness of the lips, using a soft nylon toothbrush, oral baking soda rinses and moistening food with sauces or gravies are all appropriate teaching points for patients undergoing radiation therapy to the head and neck.

8. B: The Philadelphia chromosome is present in nearly all CML cases and is detected by cytogenetic analysis. In only 5-10% of CML cases is the Philadelphia chromosome absent.

Chromosome 7 is linked to leukemias, lymphomas and MDS syndrome. Chromosome 13 is linked to retinoblastoma and other types of cancer. P53 is a tumor suppressor protein.

9. D: The TNM system for cancer staging outlined by the American Joint Committee on Cancer (AJCC) assesses three basic components: size of the primary tumor, absence or presence of regional lymph nodes and the absence or presence of distant metastatic disease. Any evidence of distant metastasis per TNM staging would classify the cancer as stage 4.

10. C: "B symptoms" associated with a lymphoma diagnosis are a key factor in the staging of the disease. The presence of B symptoms is associated with a poorer prognosis. Unexplained fever, drenching night sweats, weight loss and pruritus are all B symptoms associated with lymphoma. Headache, edema, and painful lymph nodes are not classified as B symptoms.

11. E: Vesicant chemotherapeutic agents have the potential to cause severe tissue damage if they leak into the subcutaneous tissue during an extravasation. ABVD can also cause infertility as well as birth defects. Answer B is not correct because none of the medications in ABVD are classified as monoclonal antibodies. Answer D is also not correct because ABVD will cause hair loss as a side effect.

12. D: Tyrosine kinase inhibitors are defined as antineoplastic agents that interfere with cell communication and growth through inhibition of the tyrosine kinase enzyme. Sunitinib is a tyrosine kinase inhibitor indicated in the treatment of gastrointestinal stromal tumors. Rituximab and trastuzumab are classified as monoclonal antibodies. Bortezomib is a proteasome inhibitor.

13. A: Approximately 170,000 cases of brain metastases are diagnosed in the United States each year. Although any malignancy can lead to metastasis, melanoma and lung, breast, renal, and colon cancers account for the greatest majority of brain metastases. Sixty-five percent of melanomas metastasize to the brain. Lymphoma, ovarian cancer and thyroid cancer are not common cancers with brain metastases.

14. D: Breast cancer, lymphoma, and leukemia all pose the greatest risk for the development of cardiac tamponade. This condition is an oncologic emergency with the severity dependent upon the amount of fluid in the pericardium, the rate of fluid accumulation, and the level of pericardial compromise caused by the cancer.

15. A: Several anti-emetic agents are available for use as either single agents or in combination for nausea and vomiting associated with chemotherapy administration. The oral route is the preferred route for the prophylactic treatment of nausea and vomiting. Parenteral or rectal routes are recommended if the patient is unable to keep oral medications down.

16. C: Bladder cancer is the most common malignancy of the urinary tract with a higher incidence in males versus females. Risk factors include chemical carcinogenic exposure, tobacco use, a diet high in fat, and recurrent urinary tract infections. Although all of the above symptoms may be present, gross hematuria is the most common presenting sign of bladder cancer.

17. C: Burning, frequency and urgency are common side effects from BCG treatment, therefore the answer is C. Urinalysis is performed prior to BCG treatment to look for signs of infection. The urinary catheter is clamped to hold the medication in the bladder and the patient is turned to ensure maximal bladder tissue exposure. A patient is instructed to void after catheter removal to ensure that he is able to void post-catheterization and that the urine is disposed of in a proper manner prior to the patient going home.

18. C: Radical cystectomy is the treatment of choice for bladder tumors that have invaded the surrounding muscle. Chemotherapy and radiation therapy may be viable treatment options after a surgical resection. Neither chemotherapy nor radiation therapy alone are options for invasive bladder cancer. Laser treatment would be indicated for a patient with recurrent localized disease.

19. D: Hypertension, Cushing's syndrome and non-metastatic hepatopathy are all paraneoplastic conditions associated with renal carcinomas. Additional conditions include hypercalcemia, erythrocytosis, pyrexia, galactorrhea, gynecomastia and serum glucose abnormalities. Plummer-Vinson syndrome is associated with gastric carcinomas and is characterized by weakness and difficulty swallowing due to small growths of tissue that form in the esophagus.

20. B: Renal cell carcinoma accounts for 3% of all tumors diagnosed in the United States each year. It is more prevalent in males and the etiology is unknown. Renal cell carcinomas metastasize most often to the lung (75%), soft tissues (36%), bones (20%) and liver (18%). Approximately one-third of all patients diagnosed with renal cell carcinoma have metastasis at the time of diagnosis.

21. A: The most common malignancy diagnosed in the United States is prostate cancer, with an estimated 238,000 new cases expected in 2013. It is the second leading cause of male cancer death in the United States with an increased prevalence in African American men. The median age of diagnosis for prostate cancer is 72 years, with a higher incidence occurring in each decade of life after age 50.

22. B: Strong correlations have been found between a high fat diet and the risk of prostate cancer. Dietary consumption of foods containing lycopene may decrease the risk of prostate cancer. Increasing dietary fiber may help decrease the risk by helping to lower circulating testosterone and estradiol levels. There has been no evidence to support the effect of multiple sexual partners on the development of prostate cancer.

23. B: An official diagnosis of prostate cancer has not been made, therefore the next step would be confirmation via needle biopsy. Once a diagnosis is made, treatment options can be established. Careful observation may be indicated for those with stage 1 disease. Chemotherapy and clinical trials may be options for those with advanced disease.

24. A: Radical prostatectomy is typically reserved for patients without evidence of metastatic disease. Pain management, hormonal therapy and external beam radiation therapy are all viable treatment options for patients with advanced disease or for those who are not appropriate surgical candidates.

25. D: A clinically palpable tumor confined to the prostate is indicative of a stage T2 prostate cancer per TNM staging. PIN involves ductal acinar dysplasia of the prostate and is

considered a premalignancy that can be high or low grade. Low grade PIN is associated with a lower risk of development of prostate carcinoma.

26. C: Clinical signs of neoplastic cardiac tamponade include: tachycardia, low systolic blood pressure, vasoconstriction and increased central venous pressure (CVP). As a result of increased central venous pressure, patients often experience pulsus paradoxus and jugular venous distension. A hallmark of cardiac tamponade known as Beck's triad includes an elevated CVP, distant or muffled heart sounds and arterial hypotension.

27. B: Eating a low-residue diet and maintaining adequate fluid intake may help to prevent or reduce symptoms caused by pelvic radiation therapy for prostate cancer. Radiation therapy may or may not cause erectile dysfunction, and the effects may be delayed. Sitz baths and topical hydrocortisone may be used for rectal irritation. Treatment-related side effects may involve fatigue, as well as more frequent bowel movements, urinary frequency, and mucosal bleeding.

28. A: Cabazitaxel is a taxane derivative indicated for treatment of hormone-refractory metastatic prostate cancer. Paclitaxel is not approved for this type of treatment. Sipuleucel-T is classified as an immunotherapeutic drug. Leuprolide-acetate is a gonadotropin-releasing hormone used for palliative treatment of advanced prostate cancer.

29. C: Cryptorchidism is associated with a five times greater than normal risk of testicular cancer. Research has not supported that testicular trauma, viral infections, or DES exposure before birth increase the risk of testicular cancer development.

30. D: Hematuria is a clinical feature of carcinoma of the bladder and kidneys and late stage cervical cancer. Abdominal aching, low back pain, and gynecomastia are all clinical features of testicular cancer. Patients may present with non-tender and enlarged testicles or diffuse pain and testicular swelling.

31. C: Irinotecan is indicated in the treatment of metastatic colorectal cancer. Side effects include myelosuppression, nausea, vomiting, dyspnea, and alopecia in addition to severe and potentially life-threatening diarrhea. Although the other chemotherapeutic agents listed can cause diarrhea as a side effect, dose-limiting diarrhea is a specific toxicity associated with irinotecan.

32. A: The Occupational Safety and Health Administration (OSHA) recommends the use of a disposable, long-sleeved gown, disposable gloves (non-powdered made of surgical latex, nitrile, polyurethane or neoprene), and a plastic face shield when splashes, sprays or aerosols may be generated. N95 masks are not indicated for administration. Gowns should never be reused.

33. D: Appropriate personal protective equipment is critically important in the administration of chemotherapy. Spiking and priming of hazardous drugs should be done in a biologic safety cabinet or by using a dry spike extension and backflow technique to minimize exposure.

34. A: Malignant melanoma is the most deadly form of skin cancer, accounting for 3% of all cancers diagnosed in the United States each year. Risk factors for the development of melanoma include: history of multiple blistering sun burns, blond or red hair and marked

freckling, a familial history of melanoma, the presence of atypical moles, and fair skin that burns easily. Human papillomavirus infection and excessive alcohol intake are risk factors for the development of head and neck cancers. Obesity, diabetes, and hypertension are risk factors in the development of endometrial cancer.

35. B: This patient demonstrates signs of tumor lysis syndrome as evidenced by hyperphosphatemia, hypocalcemia, and hyperkalemia. Tumor lysis syndrome is an oncologic emergency that occurs when cancer cells are rapidly killed and intracellular contents are released into the bloodstream. The patient is at risk for tumor lysis due to his diagnosis of a hematologic tumor and a large tumor burden and elevated LDH.

36. C: Disseminated intravascular coagulation is a bleeding disorder characterized by an alteration in the body's ability to clot, resulting in an abnormal acceleration of the clotting cascade and subsequent thrombosis. In DIC, excess thrombin results in multiple fibrin clots in the circulation, which trap platelets, thereby disrupting normal coagulation and decreasing the platelet count.

37. C: Septic shock is characterized by fever, chills, tachycardia, tachypnea, mental status changes and hypotension despite aggressive fluid challenge to correct the situation. The patient is not exhibiting signs of anaphylaxis or tumor lysis syndrome. Her chemotherapy was administered 10 days ago. Although the patient may be at risk for hypercalcemia, she is not exhibiting signs and symptoms of this condition either.

38. C: The cutting of cuticles is not recommended in the prevention of lymphedema. Removal of lymph nodes increases the risk for infection and lymphedema. Maintaining skin integrity helps to minimize the risk of both. Recommended interventions from the National Lymphedema Network include avoiding heavy sun exposure and burns, wearing gloves while gardening; using only the unaffected arm for injections, blood samples, intravenous access, or blood pressure readings; and promptly treating cuts.

39. B: Epidermal growth factor receptor is a protein that influences cancer growth in different types of cancers. It is found in abnormally high levels on the surface of many types of cancer cells, causing them to excessively divide in its presence. Increased EGFR is associated with more aggressive tumors, recurrence, poorer prognosis, and resistance to endocrine therapy.

40. C: Epidermal growth factor receptor inhibitors work by blocking the epidermal growth factor receptor protein present on the surface of the cancer cell that causes excessive cell division and subsequent tumor growth. Lapatinib is an epidermal growth factor receptor inhibitor used in the treatment of metastatic breast cancer. Bevacizumab is a VEGF inhibitor. Imatinib is a tyrosine kinase inhibitor. Gemtuzumab is a monoclonal antibody.

41. A: Monoclonal antibodies can be divided into two types: unconjugated and conjugated. Unconjugated monoclonal antibodies are those not bound to a drug, toxin, or radioactive substance. Unconjugated MAbs may also be referred to as naked MAbs and are the most commonly used monoclonal antibodies. Trastuzumab is an example of an unconjugated MAb. Gemtuzumab, ibritumomab, and iodine-131 tositumomab are all examples of conjugated MAbs.

42. D: Conjugated MAbs are joined to radioactive isotopes, chemotherapeutic agents, or toxins to poison the cancer cells they are targeting. Conjugated MAbs work by transporting the associated anticancer agents directly to the cancer cells. Conjugated MAbs do not attach to hormones.

43. B: Ibritumomab is indicated in combination with rituximab in the treatment of relapsed or refractory low-grade, follicular or transformed B-cell NHL. Gemtuzumab is indicated for the treatment of CD33 positive acute myeloid leukemia. Iodine-131 tositumomab is indicated for the treatment of CD20 positive, follicular NHL (not used in combination with rituximab). Alemtuzumab is indicated for the treatment of B-cell chronic lymphocytic leukemia.

44. D: Estrogen receptor-positive tumors are less likely to respond to and benefit from treatment with chemotherapy when it is used as an isolated treatment. Estrogen receptive-positive tumors are well differentiated and are more likely to respond to and benefit from endocrine therapy. Additionally, they tend to have a prolonged overall survival rate in comparison with ER-negative tumors.

45. B: Lung cancer is the leading cause of cancer deaths among women, with breast cancer being the second most common, and colorectal cancer as the third. Historically, lung cancer was more prevalent in men; however in recent years, that gap has narrowed. Tobacco use continues to account for a large proportion of lung cancers.

46. D: Anxiety occurs often in cancer patients and may be related to disease stage, treatment regimens, financial concerns, family issues, or physiological causes. It can be rated as mild, moderate or severe. Hormone-secreting tumors, hypoxia, and poorly-controlled pain are all physiologic states that can cause anxiety in patients with advanced disease.

47. C: Rapid relief of anxiety by pharmacologic intervention establishes credibility and enables the patient to discuss fears calmly. Drug therapy can be discontinued if other non-pharmacologic measures that are added afterward are successful in controlling anxiety. Relaxation techniques can be introduced once the patient's anxiety has lessened and should not be introduced while the patient is experiencing moderate or severe anxiety.

48. D: Benzodiazepines (lorazepam and midazolam) are first-line agents utilized for the treatment of anxiety and panic. Other agents, including neuroleptics (haloperidol) or anti-depressants may also be used in the treatment of anxiety. Dicyclomine is an anticholinergic agent that may produce symptoms of anxiety and is not indicated for its treatment.

49. B: Hypnotic medications prescribed in the treatment of insomnia should only be taken for short periods (less than three weeks). The lowest effective dose should be given and the patient should only use the hypnotic intermittently (2-4 times per week). Hypnotic medications should not be stopped abruptly; instead, the doses should be tapered over several days.

50. A: Approximately 85% of patients with bony metastases have a primary tumor in the breast or the prostate, and 44 % have a primary lung tumor. Patients experiencing widespread bone metastasis are likely to have a decreased survival time.

51. C: Both breast and prostate cancers have the potential to metastasize to almost anywhere in the body; however, the most common metastatic sites are the liver, lungs, brain, and bones. Skeletal metastasis commonly occurs in the vertebra, pelvis, femur and skull. Bone metastasis can be extremely painful for patients, and pain is often an initial symptom that detects when metastasis has occurred. Pain control is critical for patients with painful bone metastasis. Bone metastasis is a significant contributory factor in cancer morbidity.

52. B: Bone lesions can be classified as osteolytic, osteoblastic, or mixed. Osteolytic bone lesions are primarily associated with non-small cell lung cancer and multiple myeloma. Osteoblastic bone lesions are often associated with small cell lung cancer, prostate cancer, thyroid cancer, and Hodgkin's disease. Mixed osteolytic and osteoblastic lesions are associated with breast cancer, gastrointestinal cancers, and squamous cancers.

53. C: The treatment of choice for localized bone metastasis is external beam radiation therapy. Cox-2 inhibitors provide pain relief to patients suffering from arthritis. Chemotherapy might be used as tumor treatment, but pain control may not appear until after the tumor has been managed. Kyphoplasty can be used to treat painful compression fractures.

54. C: Bisphosphonates are often used as a preventive measure in patients with bone metastases from breast cancer or multiple myeloma. They can be given either orally or intravenously, and are effective in alleviating bone pain in both types of lesions: osteolytic and osteoblastic. Bisphosphonates are also indicated in the treatment of hypercalcemia.

55. D: Hypercalcemia is a common complication associated with malignancy and metastasis. It is considered an oncologic complication that has the potential to be life-threatening if left untreated. Breast cancer, multiple myeloma and thyroid cancer are all cancers most often associated with hypercalcemia. Prostate cancer is rarely or never associated with hypercalcemia despite a high frequency of bone metastases.

56. C: Neoplastic fever is defined as a fever caused by the cancer itself and is believed to be cytokine mediated. Cytokines stimulate the production of prostaglandins that act on the hypothalamus, creating a rise in body temperature. Neoplastic fever is the most common cause of fever of unknown origin in cancer patients.

57. B: Pruritus is associated with chronic renal failure, obstructive hepatobiliary disease, Hodgkin's disease, cutaneous infiltration of malignancy, hyperthyroidism, polycythemia vera and iron deficiency. It is a "B" symptom present in Hodgkin's disease. Pruritus occurs in 90% of dialysis patients and is not dose-related to the bilirubin level in obstructive hepatobiliary disease.

58. C: Biliary stent failure most often occurs around 4.5 months after stent placement. Fever, chills, sweating, pruritus, return of jaundice, abdominal pain, dark urine, and pale stools are all signs of stent failure. If stent failure is suspected, it must be properly managed as sepsis may occur if the blocked stent is not promptly replaced.

59. D: Persistent or intractable hiccups may be caused by irritation of the vagus or phrenic nerves due to tumors of the neck, lung, or mediastinum. Pharmacologic agents such as IV corticosteroids, barbiturates, or benzodiazepines can also cause intractable hiccups. Gastric

distension due to impaired gastric motility is a potential cause as well. Hyponatremia may develop when a patient with polydipsia attempts to relieve hiccups, however, hyponatremia itself will not cause intractable hiccups.

60. A: Nausea and vomiting occur in up to 60% of patients receiving opioids, especially at the initiation of treatment. Nausea and vomiting occur in approximately 40% of patients during their last week of life, and tend to be more prevalent in patients with breast, stomach, and gynecologic cancers. Drug therapy is more likely to succeed if given prophylactically.

61. B: A ceiling effect occurs when, after a certain dosage of medication is given, increasing the dosage will not produce further analgesia. This is true of all non-opioid medications. A synergistic effect of a medication is defined as enhancing the action of another medication. An analgesic effect is defined as relieving pain. An antagonistic effect is defined as having an opposite effect on the body when two drugs are given in combination.

62. C: Nociceptive or somatic pain is defined as pain resulting from stimulation of afferent nerves, connective tissue, muscles, joints, or bones. It is usually localized and described as throbbing, sharp, or aching. Neuropathic pain is related to damage to the nervous system (i.e. peripheral neuropathy). Breakthrough pain occurs intermittently, is of rapid onset, and greater in intensity than baseline pain. Idiopathic pain is defined as pain that has no apparent underlying cause.

63. B: Bone metastases are examples of nociceptive pain. Diabetic neuropathy and complex regional pain syndrome are examples of neuropathic pain. Fibromyalgia is an example of idiopathic pain. Nociceptive pain is the type of pain related to bone, soft tissue, or internal organ damage and usually presents as a throbbing, sharp, or aching pain.

64. A: Double effect is defined as the difference between providing analgesic medication with the intent to relieve pain that might inadvertently hasten death versus providing medication to intentionally cause death. An effect arising between two or more medications that produce an effect greater than the sum of the two is a synergistic effect. Tolerance or resistance to a drug that develops through continued use of another drug with similar pharmacologic action is defined as cross tolerance.

65. D: The World Health Organization has defined the principles of managing pain in cancer patients as the following: By mouth: the oral route is the choice route of administration. By the clock: analgesics for moderate to severe pain should be given on a fixed dose schedule around the clock and not on an "as needed" basis. By the ladder: the WHO has developed a three-step analgesic ladder to guide the sequential use of drugs in treating cancer pain. By the diagnosis is not a principle included in the WHO definition of pain management principles.

66. C: Carbamazepine used in combination with an opioid is useful in the treatment of neuropathic pain. Codeine, in combination with a non-steroid anti-inflammatory agent, may be useful for visceral pain. Dexamethasone in higher doses is useful in the treatment of increased intracranial pressure. Diazepam may be utilized in treating muscle spasms.

67. D: Many patients have misconceptions regarding morphine and other narcotics. Fear that morphine causes significant respiratory depression is common. When morphine is

titrated according to a patient's pain, the pain antagonizes morphine's depressant effects. Significant respiratory depression is not commonly seen in cancer patients when the medication is appropriately titrated. Common side effects such as nausea, dizziness, and sleepiness are often misinterpreted by patients as an allergic response. There is no evidence suggesting that dose-appropriate morphine either hastens death or prolongs life. The patient recognizing that he may require more morphine as his disease progresses demonstrates an understanding of the medication. Additionally, morphine has no analgesic ceiling; therefore a dose adjustment based on the patient's pain may be beneficial.

68. D: The effect of opioids on the GI system include a decrease in intestinal secretions and peristalsis. Opioids affect GI function by increasing muscle tone in the gastric antrum, small intestine, and colon; increasing segmental contractions of the bowel, decreasing stool volume and frequency, and increasing water and electrolyte absorption from the gut lumen.

69. A: Ascites is defined as an excessive accumulation of fluid between the abdominal lining and the peritoneal cavity. Ascites can affect comfort level, mobility, respiratory effort, and activities of daily living. Ovarian cancer is the most common malignancy associated with ascites, and 35% of patients will have ascites upon diagnosis. Sixty percent will have ascites at the time of death.

70. C: Peritoneal carcinomatosis is the most common cause of ascites in cancer patients. Tumor invasion of liver parenchyma only accounts for around 15% of ascites cases. Bulging flanks may become apparent when there is more than 500-1000 ml of fluid in the abdomen. Up to 65% of patients will respond to diuretics. Paracentesis may be considered in those patients with tense ascites or ascites that causes distressing symptoms.

71. A: Brain metastases occur in 25-35% of all cancer patients. They most commonly occur in patients with lung cancer, followed by breast cancer and melanoma. Brain metastases are more common than primary brain tumors and are multiple in 60% of cases.

72. D: Clinical features of patients with brain metastases may include headache, weakness, seizures, blurred vision, gait disturbance, altered sensation, and changes in personality. The most common presenting symptom is a headache. Ataxia is often seen with cerebellar metastases, occurring in 24% of diagnosed patients. Seizures occur in 15% of patients and focal weakness in 40%.

73. D: Seizure activity is seen in 20-50% of all patients with brain tumors; however, seizures may occur in patients with advanced cancer as a result of stroke, pre-existing seizure disorder, hypoxemia, hypoglycemia, uremia, hyponatremia, sepsis, or withdrawal from drugs or alcohol. Increased intracranial pressure may also result in seizure activity in cancer patients.

74. B: Different performance scales exist that assess patient well-being and quality of life. The Karnofsky Performance Scale allows patients to be classified as to their functional impairment. The lower the Karnofsky score, the worse the survival for most serious illnesses. It is an effective means of comparing different therapies and assessing the prognosis of individual patients.

75. C: It may be difficult to diagnose depression in the patient with advanced cancer, as many physical signs of depression are similar to those caused by the cancer itself. Weight

loss, insomnia, and diminished concentration are all somatic symptoms of depression that may also be present because of cancer. Feelings of worthlessness are psychological symptoms of depression that may aid in diagnosis when present.

76. C: A sexual health assessment should be obtained early in the nurse-patient relationship to set the expectation that sexuality is an important component of good health. The assessment should begin with less-sensitive topics and move to more sensitive issues throughout the assessment. It is important to assess the patient's goals for treatment as well as the impact treatment could have on the patient's sexuality. Once goals of treatment are assessed, the nurse can explore any sexuality concerns that the patient may have in regard to his treatment.

77. A: In the PLISSIT model often utilized for sexuality counseling, the "P" stands for permission. Obtaining permission as a first step in the process promotes discussion and allowance of the patient and his/her partner to speak openly without embarrassment. The PLISSIT model can be utilized to guide the nurse in performing a sexuality assessment as well as a means to incorporate nursing interventions based on the nurse's knowledge and comfort level.

78. B: Asking the patient how he is able to discuss his illness with his support system is a suitable way to help facilitate discussion and assist the patient in finding meaning in his illness. Comparing the patient to other cancer patients or making assumptions as to why the patient feels the way he does are not therapeutic communication options that would allow the patient to feel comfortable discussing his feelings.

79. C: An allogeneic bone marrow transplant is a transplant in which the patient receives someone else's bone marrow. Syngeneic allogeneic transplants occur when the donor is the patient's identical twin. Related allogeneic transplants occur when the donor is related to the recipient (usually a sibling). Unrelated transplants occur when the donor is of no relation to the recipient. An autologous transplant is a transplant in which the patient's own bone marrow is used.

80. C: A dental consult, hepatitis screen, and ABO and Rh typing are all routine tests that are generally required for a patient to complete prior to having a bone marrow transplant. PET scans are performed to detect, stage, and evaluate recurrence of cancer and are not a routine part of a pre-transplantation evaluation.

81. B: Radiation pneumonitis is a complication of radiation therapy that is dependent on the dose of radiation administered. It can occur 3-24 weeks after therapy and the patient may present with dyspnea, a hacking cough, chest pain, fever, and night sweats. The hallmark treatment of radiation pneumonitis is steroid therapy. Radiation pneumonitis is dose limiting if it develops while the patient is undergoing radiation therapy.

82. C: The process by which normal cells are transformed into cancer cells is known as carcinogenesis. Metastasis is defined as the spread of cancer from one part of the body to another. Carcinomatosis is a condition that occurs when cancer spreads widely throughout the body, often encompassing a large region. Meiosis is a form of cell division where each daughter cell receives half the amount of DNA as the parent cell. Meiosis occurs during the formation of egg and sperm cells.

83. D: Medicare provides coverage for hospice care to individual patients who are entitled to Part A Medicare coverage and who have been certified as terminally ill with a prognosis for a life expectancy of six months or less. The patient or their authorized representative must elect hospice care in order to receive it. Only a medical doctor or a doctor of osteopathic medicine can certify or re-certify a terminal illness. The certification must contain a statement of the patient's prognosis and life expectancy of less than six months, a brief narrative explaining the clinical findings and how they relate to the patient's prognosis, and the benefit period dates that the certification covers.

84. C: Palliative sedation therapy is defined as the use of sedative medications to relieve intractable symptoms for patients with irreversible and terminal disease. Patients who do not have a terminal disease are not candidates for palliative sedation therapy. Patients must have a do-not-resuscitate order in place and indications for the initiation of palliative sedation. It is important that the patient, family, and staff recognize that palliative sedation is not the same as passive euthanasia. The goal of palliative sedation is to manage intractable symptoms and not hasten death. Palliative sedation therapy should be only performed in the presence of a physician.

85. A: Anti-metabolites are cell-cycle phase specific and include drugs such as cytarabine and 5-flourouracil. Anti-metabolites work by blocking essential enzymes that are necessary for DNA synthesis. Antitumor antibiotics are cell-cycle phase non-specific and work by disrupting DNA transcription and inhibiting DNA and RNA synthesis. Alkylating agents are cell-cycle phase non-specific and work by forming a molecular bond with nucleic acids, interfering with nucleic acid duplication and preventing mitosis. Nitrosoureas are also cell-cycle phase non-specific. Their action is similar to that of alkylating agents in that the synthesis of both DNA and RNA is inhibited.

86. D: The emetogenic potential of chemotherapeutic agents can be classified as mild, moderate, or severe. Cisplatin is classified as an agent with severe emetogenic potential and often causes delayed or persistent nausea and vomiting. Paclitaxel is classified as a chemotherapeutic drug with mild emetogenic potential. Carboplatin and cytarabine are both classified as agents with moderate emetogenic potential. Cytarabine and carboplatin can also cause neurotoxicity and myelosuppression.

87. C: Acupuncture is an alternative therapy that has been utilized in the United States for over 200 years. It involves the use of needles, heat, and pressure to various points on the skin. Acupuncture is used to treat symptoms caused by many illnesses, including cancer. Clinical trials have supported the effectiveness of acupuncture in relieving nausea and vomiting caused by chemotherapy. Acupuncture should be performed by a qualified professional who uses clean, disposable needles for each patient. Infections are not likely to be a complication if clean needles are used. Many patients elect to pursue alternative therapies in addition to conventional treatments. Nurses should remain free from judgment regarding alternative therapies and be able to provide clarifying information about such therapies.

88. C: In Phase 3 of a clinical trial, the overall benefit versus the risk of the drug is evaluated and more data regarding safety and efficacy is established. Phase 1 has a primary focus on patient safety and is the phase in which the maximum tolerated dose is determined. The most frequent and serious adverse effects are recorded as well as how the drug is metabolized and excreted. Phase 1 clinical trials work to establish an effective drug

administration schedule. Phase 2 is where the preliminary data on the drug's effectiveness is established. Short-term adverse reactions are studied. Phase 4 occurs after the drug has been approved by the FDA for marketing purposes. Additional information regarding safety and efficacy are established, with the goal of refining the protocol to determine the optimal treatment use of the new drug.

89. D: Cancer cells possess many characteristics that make them unique. Proliferation is uncontrolled in cancer cells and there is an imbalance between cell production and cell loss. Control mechanisms that exist in normal cells fail with cancer cells, resulting in uncontrolled growth. Differentiation occurs when cells "diversify" and gain specific structural and functional characteristics. In cancer cells, differentiation refers to how comparable the cancer cells are to normal cells. Well-differentiated cancer cells look the most like normal cells. Poorly- differentiated cells or undifferentiated cells have lost the capacity for specialized functions. The more undifferentiated the cell is, the poorer the prognosis. Cancer cells are less stable genetically than normal cells. Chromosomal instability causes new malignant mutant cells that have the ability to survive despite therapy. Cancer cells have the ability to become increasingly malignant and metastasize.

90. B: B-cell lymphoma is the most frequently diagnosed malignancy in patients infected with HIV. HIV-related lymphoma is most likely to present as a B-cell tumor of intermediate or high-grade histologic type. Since the use of highly active antiretroviral therapy (HAART), the incidence of Kaposi's sarcoma has declined significantly among HIV patients. Although HIV-infected patients have been diagnosed with multiple myeloma and B-cell acute lymphocytic leukemia, no causal relationship has been identified.

91. C: Fatigue is the most frequently-experienced symptom of cancer and accompanies most malignancies. Chemotherapy, immunotherapy, and radiation therapy are all contributing factors that increase fatigue in cancer patients. Fatigue caused by radiation therapy affects almost 100% of patients and is cumulative in nature over the course of treatment. Cancer-related anemia is also a contributing factor. It is important for the oncology nurse to recognize that fatigue is a "self-recognized" state in which the patient experiences an overwhelming and sustained sense of exhaustion not relieved by rest.

92. B: Hormonal therapy can cause several side effects impacting a patient's sexual function and fertility. Patients on hormonal agents should avoid becoming pregnant during treatment and for at least two months post-treatment due to increased risk of adverse fetal effects. Hormonal therapy may cause decreased vaginal lubrication, changes in sexuality, masculinization, amenorrhea or oligomenorrhea, vaginal bleeding or discharge, mood swings, hot flashes, sleep disturbances, and dyspareunia. Patients receiving hormonal therapy should be educated on these side effects and the potential impact on sexual function.

93. A: Bevacizumab is a humanized MAb and vascular endothelial growth factor inhibitor used in the treatment of metastatic colorectal cancer. There is a greater risk of impaired wound healing and surgical complications among patients who are receiving bevacizumab. Due to the potential complications with wound healing, bevacizumab should not be given for at least 28 days following major surgery or until the wound is healed.

94. D: Cancer survival begins when a patient is first diagnosed and continues through treatment, remission, recurrence, and the final stages of life up to and including death.

There are three stages of survival: acute, extended, and permanent. Survivorship includes physiologic, psychologic, social, and spiritual effects. Survivorship issues affect others, not just the cancer survivor. Family, friends, significant others, and co-workers are also affected and are considered "secondary survivors."

95. C: Absent grief occurs when the patient appears to act as if nothing has happened. Often times, he will not speak of or permit any reference to the deceased. Absent grief can lead to clinical depression and may manifest itself through physical symptoms. Chronic and conflicted grief are types of pathologic grieving that warrant further follow up by the health care team. Chronic grief continues and does not wane in intensity. The bereaved person often gets stuck in a particular stage of grieving and cannot move forward. In conflicted grief, the bereaved person has unresolved feelings of ambivalence toward the deceased that result in feelings of anger and guilt.

96. A: Ipilimumab is a monoclonal antibody that is FDA-approved for the treatment of unresectable or metastatic melanoma. The FDA has a Risk Evaluation and Mitigation Strategy (REMS) program in place to ensure the benefits of treatment outweigh the risk. Treatment with ipilimumab can result in severe and fatal immune-mediated adverse reactions as a result of T-cell activation and proliferation. The most common manifestations of these reactions include enterocolitis, hepatitis, dermatitis, neuropathy, and endocrinopathy. Hypotension can occur as part of the endocrine immune-mediated adverse reaction. Vasculitis and autoimmune thyroiditis are clinically significant immune-mediated adverse reactions that may result in discontinuation of therapy but are less likely to be severe or fatal in nature.

97. D: Carfilzomib is a proteasome inhibitor indicated in the treatment of relapsed or refractory multiple myeloma. Carfilzomib is indicated for patients who have received at least two prior therapies including bortezomib and an immunomodulatory agent and have experienced disease progression on or within 60 days of completion of therapy. Omalizumab is a monoclonal antibody used in the treatment of moderate to severe persistent asthma. Lapatinib is both a tyrosine kinase inhibitor and an epidermal growth factor inhibitor, used in the treatment of metastatic breast cancer. Thalidomide is an angiogenesis inhibitor often used in combination with chemotherapy for the treatment of multiple myeloma.

98. D: Chemotherapy-induced peripheral neuropathy (CIPN) is a common side effect that often causes both physical and emotional symptoms. Healthcare providers must be diligent and proactive in their assessment of CIPN. Patients receiving chemotherapy should be assessed for CIPN at every visit. Upper extremity symptoms, although not as common as deficits in the lower extremities, affect the fine motor skills, including difficulties with buttoning or zipping clothing, poor grip strength, and problems with handwriting. Physical and occupational therapies should be included in the treatment plan for those patients experiencing CIPN causing physical limitations.

99. B: Tamoxifen is indicated as adjuvant hormonal therapy for the treatment of hormone-sensitive breast cancer in pre-menopausal women. Although depression can be a side effect of tamoxifen therapy, the occurrence is only 2-12%. Bupropion is a strong inhibitor of CYP2D6, which can adversely affect the success of the tamoxifen in preventing breast cancer recurrence. Strong inhibitors of CYP2D6 such as bupropion, paroxetine and fluoxetine should be avoided in patients receiving tamoxifen. Other anti-depressant medications

should be considered instead.

100. C: Clinical manifestations of multiple myeloma include hyperkalemia, renal insufficiency, anemia and bone lesions. Lab studies may show anemia, thrombocytopenia, leucopenia, and elevated blood urea nitrogen levels. Anorexia may be present along with weakness, weight loss, and fatigue. Pain is more likely to be associated with bone lesions and may present as back pain, rather than abdominal pain.

101. B: The effects of surviving a cancer diagnosis can be categorized as physiologic, psychologic, social, and spiritual. These effects can occur at any point across the survivorship continuum. Ambivalence regarding health care follow up is an example of a psychologic effect that may occur in cancer survivors. Peripheral neuropathy is an example of a physiologic effect that can occur as a result of cancer treatment. Fears regarding employment, including the fear of loss of employment, loss of benefits, and lack of promotion are examples of social effects that may occur. Cancer survivors may experience spiritual effects from having experienced cancer, including an increased passion and zest for life or increased self-acceptance.

102. C: According to the National Cancer Institute, cancer survivors have a 14% higher risk of developing a new cancer. The development of a secondary cancer is most likely caused by previous cancer treatments including chemotherapy, radiation therapy, and bone marrow and stem cell transplants. Patients should be educated to discuss risk-lowering strategies with their physician and how to watch for signs and symptoms of a secondary malignancy.

103. D: Possible long-term or late side effects can occur in patients treated for cancer. Secondary cancers, fertility issues; and thyroid, heart, and lung problems are among the possible long-term effects a patient may experience after undergoing treatment for Hodgkin's disease. The ABVD regimen, a common treatment for Hodgkin's disease, contains the drug bleomycin, which can cause irreversible damage to the lungs. If the patient received radiation therapy to the chest, lung damage may also occur. The patient complaining of shortness of breath post treatment should be further evaluated to determine the cause.

104. B: Pertuzumab is a humanized monoclonal antibody that targets extracellular human epidermal growth factor receptor 2 protein. It is used in combination with trastuzumab and docetaxel for the treatment of metastatic breast cancer in patients who have not received prior anti-HER2 therapy or chemotherapy to treat metastatic disease. When combined with trastuzumab, a more complete inhibition of HER 2 signaling occurs due to the binding of pertuzumab to a different isotope than trastuzumab.

105. B: According to the common terminology criteria for adverse effects developed by the National Cancer Institute and National Institute of Health, Mr. Smith's constipation would be classified as a Grade 2. Grade 2 constipation is defined as persistent symptoms with regular use of laxatives or enemas and limiting instrumental activities of daily living. Grade 1 is defined as occasional or intermittent symptoms with occasional use of stool softeners or laxatives. Grade 3 is defined as obstipation with manual evacuation indicated. Grade 4 has life-threatening consequences with urgent intervention needed.

106. C: Mrs. Jones' neuropathy would fall into the Grade 3 category, which is defined as severe symptoms that limit self-care activities of daily living. Grade 1 peripheral neuropathy

- 46 -

per the NCI grading scale is defined as a loss of deep tendon reflexes or paresthesia with the patient being asymptomatic. Grade 2 neuropathy is defined as moderate symptoms with limitations on instrumental ADL's. Grade 4 is defined as having life-threatening consequences with urgent intervention needed.

107. B: The National Cancer Institute (NCI) created a Common Toxicity Criteria system (CTC v 1.0) in 1983 to aid in the recognition and grading of adverse effects of chemotherapy. This system was revised in 2006 and represents the first comprehensive, multimodality grading system for reporting both acute and late effects of cancer treatment. The World Health Organization and Cooperative Oncology Groups also offer criteria for grading toxicities. The purpose of grading toxicities is to provide an objective assessment. The grade of toxicity will determine the reason for dosage adjustments or delays. Most toxicity scales range from 0-4, with 0 meaning no toxicity and 4 indicating severe or life-threatening toxicity or even death.

108. C: Research supports that dehydration in dying patients can actually be beneficial in alleviating symptoms such as pulmonary secretions and congestion, vomiting, edema, and ascites. Families are often troubled by the thought of their loved one experiencing dehydration and feeling thirsty. Providing the family with education regarding the benefits of dehydration in the dying patient may help to alleviate their anxiety.

109. B: Thrombotic thrombocytopenia purpura (TTP) is a blood disorder that leads to blood clots forming in small vessels throughout the body. TTP is characterized by thrombocytopenia, hemolytic anemia, and the presence of petechiae or purpura (small red or purple spots caused by hemorrhaging of small blood vessels). Patients with TTP often present with nausea, abdominal pain, fever, and fatigue. Hemoglobinuria may be present as well. Patients with a cancer diagnosis and those treated with chemotherapy may be at risk for developing TTP. Von Willebrand disease affects clotting due to a deficiency of Von Willebrand factor. Disseminated intravascular coagulation (DIC) is a bleeding disorder characterized by an alteration in the blood-clotting mechanism causing an acceleration of the clotting cascade. Hemorrhage occurs due to the depletion of clotting factors.

110. A: Thrombocytopenia is defined as a decrease in the number of circulating platelets. Leukopenia is defined as a reduction in white blood cells. Neutropenia is defined as a decrease in the number of circulating neutrophils, usually less than 1000/mm3. Anemia is defined as a decrease in hemoglobin level or circulating erythrocytes. Pancytopenia is a term used when there is a deficiency of all the cell elements of the blood including erythrocytes, platelets, and all of the components of the white blood cells.

111. C: Alteration in body image is a common occurrence among cancer patients due to the actual or perceived changes in their bodies. Nurses should be aware of this risk and assist in providing interventions to minimize the severity. Allowing patients to discuss the changes and how they are affecting them both physically and emotionally is an important aspect in helping patients to cope. False reassurance and minimization of patient feelings should be avoided. Multiple resources exist that can help patients cope with changes. Nurses should support patients through active listening and non-judgmental acceptance while allowing patients to express their feelings and grieve their losses.

112. D: In order for patient education to be effective, the nurse must evaluate and assess the patient to determine the most appropriate method of providing education. In addition to assessing the patient's learning style and potential barriers to learning, the nurse must look

at factors such as the patient's readiness and motivation to learn, his cognitive ability, and his comfort level. A person who is experiencing pain or distress will not have the ability to focus on the education provided. It is important for the nurse to ensure that the material provided is appropriate for the patient's cognitive ability. Asking the patient how they would prefer to learn will provide the nurse with options for individualizing the education plan.

113. A: High doses of opioids along with impaired renal function can cause the accumulation of opioid metabolites, resulting in hallucinations, myoclonus, and seizures. Myoclonus is defined as the involuntary jerking of a muscle or group of muscles. Myoclonus can be treated with the use of benzodiazepines. Because the dying patient has diminished renal function, less of the opioid may be needed to achieve adequate pain relief. Alteration in renal sufficiency causes less drug clearance and more of the drug and its metabolites to remain in circulation.

114. B: The Patient Self-Determination Act was passed by Congress in 1990 and requires all health care agencies including hospitals, long-term care facilities, and home health agencies that are receiving Medicare and Medicaid reimbursement to recognize living wills and durable power of attorney for health care. In addition, these facilities must ask about the presence of advanced directives at the time of admission and give patients requesting information about advance directives the appropriate information.

115. D: Interferon alpha-2 B can cause hepatotoxicity as well as hypertriglyceridemia. A normal triglyceride level is less than 150 mg/dl with levels of 500 mg/dl or higher considered in the very high range. If hypertriglyceridemia remains persistent and severe, treatment with interferon should be discontinued. Other side effects of interferon alpha-2 B include flu-like symptoms such as fever, myalgia and fatigue. Interferon can also cause neutropenia, anemia, and thrombocytopenia. Hematologic effects should be monitored and dosages adjusted or held according to severity.

116. C: A histone deacetylase inhibitor (HDACi) is a targeted therapy agent that affects cancer cells by arresting the cell cycle and inhibiting angiogenesis and cell apoptosis. Histone deacetylase inhibitors are targeted specifically toward cancer cells and appear to have little effect on normal cells due to the increased expression of HDAC in cancer cells. Currently there are two HDACi that are approved by the FDA: vorinostat and romidepsin. These drugs are approved for the treatment of cutaneous T-cell lymphoma. Romidepsin has an additional FDA approval for the treatment of peripheral T-cell lymphoma.

117. C: Totect is FDA approved for the treatment of anthracycline extravasation and has a 98% efficacy rate with minimal toxicities. Totect infusion should be initiated as soon as possible, within six hours of extravasation. Totect is administered as a three-day infusion and is given over 1-2 hours. It should be infused in an area other than the extravasation site. Ice should be applied prior to infusion and removed 15 minutes before the Totect infusion to allow sufficient blood flow to the area to maximize the ability of the drug to reach the extravasation site.

118. D: Acute myeloid leukemia (AML) is a cancer of the blood and bone marrow affecting the myeloid cells, which develop into mature blood cells, such as white cells, red cells and platelets. There are several risk factors identified in the development of acute myeloid leukemia including certain genetic disorders such as Down syndrome, Klinefelter's

syndrome and Fanconi's anemia. Additionally, previous cancer treatment, exposure to ionizing radiation, increasing age, smoking, and obesity are all believed to increase the risk of AML. Males are more likely to develop AML than females.

119. B: The most common cause of increased intracranial pressure is brain metastasis, in which vasogenic cerebral edema allows fluid and protein to leak out of the capillaries into the extracellular space, primarily in the white matter of the brain. If severe, increased intracranial pressure can displace brain tissue from one cranial compartment to another, causing herniation. Symptoms of increased intracranial pressure include headache, nausea, vomiting, change in level of consciousness, personality changes, ataxia, and seizures. Treatment should focus on the rapid reduction of cerebral edema and reduction of intracranial pressure. Corticosteroids are first line treatment that can rapidly decrease cerebral edema. Lumbar puncture should be avoided due to the risk of exacerbation and herniation. The nausea the patient is experiencing is due to the increased intracranial pressure, so a CT scan of the chest and abdomen is not indicated. Anticonvulsants can be given to manage seizures when appropriate.

120. C: Mucositis is a biologic response of the gastrointestinal mucosa to chemotherapy, radiation therapy, or bone marrow transplantation that results in inflammation and ulceration of the gastrointestinal mucosa. It can occur anywhere along the digestive tract from the mouth to the anus. It is the most debilitating symptom reported by cancer patients and it occurs in 20-40% of patients receiving chemotherapy. Patients who develop mucositis should be educated to clean their mouths with a soft toothbrush and use fluoride toothpaste. Patients who regularly floss should continue to floss unless they experience uncontrolled bleeding, have a platelet count of less than $20,000/mm^3$ or an absolute neutrophil count of less than $1000/mm^3$.

121. D: Under the Hospice Medicare Benefit, all services provided to manage symptoms related to a terminal illness are covered including: physician care, nursing care, medical equipment and supplies, medications for symptom control, home health and homemaker service; physical, occupational, and speech therapy; social work, dietary counseling, grief and loss counseling, short term inpatient and respite care, and volunteer services. Those services not covered include treatment intended to cure the illness, prescription medications to cure the illness rather than to provide symptom control, and room and board.

122. C: Communicating with terminally ill patients regarding prognosis and end of life can be difficult for health care providers. Establishing a trusting relationship with the patient is the key to effective communication. Health care providers often use medical language that can be confusing or misinterpreted by patients. Statements such as "there is nothing more that can be done" may cause patients to become fearful and feel abandoned. Active listening and responding through encouraging the patient to speak openly, summarizing the patient's message to ensure understanding, and allowing silence so the patient has time to think and respond are all strategies that can be utilized to promote effective communication.

123. D: Capecitabine is an oral antimetabolite used in the treatment of metastatic breast and colorectal cancers. It is converted to 5-flourouracil in the liver and tissues. It is administered in two divided doses 12 hours apart and should be taken within ½ hour after eating. Capecitabine should be taken at the same time each day with prescribed antiemetics. Patients should not double a dose if missed. Acute and potentially life-threatening diarrhea

can occur, so patients should be educated to notify the health care team with persistent diarrhea. Capecitabine can also cause photosensitivity, so sun exposure should be avoided.

124. C: Quadrivalent human papillomavirus recombinant vaccine (Gardasil) is indicated for the prevention of human papillomavirus-associated diseases including cervical cancer, genital warts, vulvar neoplasia, and vaginal neoplasia. It is not 100% reliable in the prevention of cervical cancer and does not protect against all causes of gynecological malignancies or sexually transmitted infections. Patients must be between the ages of 9 and 26 years of age to receive Gardasil and no pretreatment laboratory tests are required. The drug is administered as an IM injection and given in three separate doses.

125. A: Veno-occlusive disease of the liver is a life-threatening complication that occurs in 15-20% of hematopoietic stem cell transplant patients. It occurs when fibrous material accumulates, resulting in obstruction of venules in the liver, which in turn causes portal hypertension and destruction of the liver cells. Clinical manifestations include hyperbilirubinemia, weight gain, ascites, right upper quadrant pain, hepatomegaly, splenomegaly, and jaundice. Veno-occlusive disease is treated by maintaining intravascular volume and renal perfusion and minimizing fluid accumulation.

126. C: Massage therapy has many benefits in improving the health and well-being of cancer patients. The American Cancer Society has recognized the benefits of massage therapy and has recommended it as a complementary therapy for cancer patients due to its physical and psychological benefits. It is recommended that massage near tumor sites be avoided; however, research is needed to determine whether tissue manipulation from massage therapy increases the risk of metastasis. Massage therapy can improve muscle tone and mobility and can help alleviate muscular pain.

127. B: Genetic predisposition to cancer is a result of an alteration in a proto-oncogene, tumor suppressor gene, or DNA repair gene that increases a cell's susceptibility to mutate and become cancerous. Inherited cancers account for 1% of all cancers. There are over 20 hereditary cancer syndromes that have been identified including familial adenomatous polyposis, familial melanoma, and familial breast cancer. Familial cancers can be limited to a particular type of cancer or they may cause different types of cancers. Inheriting one mutated gene is usually not enough to cause cancer.

128. C: Syndrome of inappropriate antidiuretic hormone secretion (SIADH) can occur when excessive amounts of antidiuretic hormone are produced by tumor cells, resulting in excessive water retention and decreased serum sodium. SIADH occurs in 1-2% of cancer patients, with small cell lung cancer accounting for 80% of all cases. Symptoms include thirst, mild nausea and vomiting, weight gain, weakness, lethargy, confusion, and oliguria. For moderately severe hyponatremia, fluid should be restricted to 500 ml/24 hours if serum sodium level is less than 125 mEq/L. For sodium levels less than 115, 3% saline may be given along with furosemide 40-80 mg IV every 6-8 hours. Mild hyponatremia may be treated with isotonic saline or oral salt tablets. It is not recommended to correct sodium levels by more than 12 mEq/L per day.

129. D: Beginning at age 50, screening for colorectal cancer should include one of the following examination schedules: a fecal occult blood test or fecal immunochemical test every year, a flexible sigmoidoscopy every five years, a double-contrast barium enema every five years, or a colonoscopy every 10 years. Combined testing is the preferred

screening option. High-risk patients may have a different testing schedule and should discuss alternatives with their physician.

130. D: There are multiple factors that influence the grieving process. It is important as a health care provider to assess these factors and to be able to identify when the grieving individual presents with risk factors for a poor outcome. Determinants of grief include the relationship with the deceased and characteristics of the deceased, the type and length of illness as well as the mode of death, history of coping, psychological history of functioning, number and type of previous losses; social, cultural, religious, and spiritual factors; level of support, concurrent crises, and physiologic factors.

131. D: Terminal agitation is a form of delirium characterized by restlessness, anguish, and cognitive failure. Terminal agitation can be caused by an array of factors including constipation, urinary retention, high dose opioid treatment, dyspnea, hypercalcemia, medication side effects, pain, hypoglycemia, fever, anxiety, environmental stimuli, metabolic abnormalities and liver or renal failure. Terminal agitation can be further compounded by multisystem failure, poly-pharmacy; and physical, emotional, spiritual, and psychological factors. Assessment should include identification of the underlying cause and subsequent treatment.

132. A: The pre-active phase of dying occurs 7-14 days prior to death. Characteristics that patients may exhibit in this phase include progressive weakness and lethargy, increased dependence on caregivers, bedbound status in a patient who was formerly active, increased sleep, progressive disorientation, limited attention span or withdrawal, restlessness, decreased interest in food or fluid, difficulty swallowing, and loss of bladder or bowel control in previously continent patients. The active phase of dying occurs 2-3 days prior to death. Patients in this phase may experience decreased responsiveness to external stimuli, no interest in food or fluids, abnormal respiratory patterns, hypotension, progressive cooling and mottling of the extremities, and terminal congestion.

133. D: Dyspnea occurs in up to 70% of dying patients, with the highest incidence occurring in patients with lung cancer, head and neck cancer, and degenerative neurologic disease. Several non-pharmacologic treatment options exist to help alleviate and manage the associated symptoms. Presence of a caregiver, use of a soothing voice, gentle touch, relaxation techniques, circulation of air through the use of a fan or open window, and repositioning the patient to an upright position are all interventions that may help minimize the symptoms and provide patient comfort.

134. D: Mucositis, xerostomia, radiation dental caries, and osteoradionecrosis are all potential complications of radiation therapy for head and neck cancer patients. Dysgeusia may return within 4-12 months of treatment, however some patients may experience a permanent alteration. Patients experiencing xerostomia should drink plenty of water and sugar-free beverages throughout the day and may moisten food with gravies and sauces. Synthetic saliva may be used for palliation of xerostomia and lips may be moistened with lanolin or cocoa butter. Steroid creams or rinses should be avoided due to the potential to encourage oral fungal growth. Alcohol-based commercial-brand mouthwashes should be avoided due to the potential to irritate mucous membranes.

135. D: Ovarian cancer accounts for approximately 23% of all gynecologic cancers, with the majority of ovarian tumors being epithelial neoplasms. Research shows that endocrine,

environmental, and genetic factors may all play a role in the development of epithelial ovarian cancer. Risk factors include nulliparity, family history, genetic mutations including BRCA1, BRCA II, and hereditary non-polyposis colon cancer; early menarche, late menopause, white race, increasing age, and residence in Western industrialized countries.

136. B: Pegfilgrastim is a granulocyte colony stimulating factor used in reducing the incidence of febrile neutropenia for cancer patients receiving marrow toxic chemotherapeutic regimens. Pegfilgrastim is the pegylated form of filgrastim. A glycol molecule bound to filgrastim allows for reduced renal clearance of the drug, resulting in an increased half-life and single dose administration. Due to the prolonged half-life, pegfilgrastim should not be administered within the 14 days leading up to chemotherapy administration.

137. C: Dietary supplements may be helpful as a supportive measure for patients undergoing cancer treatment. Caution should be used with some dietary supplements, as many have untoward side effects and may interact with conventional therapies. Patients should always be advised to consult their physician prior to starting a supplement. Antioxidants have the potential to interfere with cancer treatment by blocking the therapeutic effects of cancer treatment. Research indicates that antioxidants may protect tumor cells in addition to protecting normal cells. Flaxseed is an herbal supplement that has been found to lower cholesterol, enhance the immune system, and prevent cancer. Ginger is an herbal supplement that has found to be useful in treating nausea and vomiting associated with chemotherapy.

138. D: Sodium thiosulfate is an antidote used in the management of extravasation of alkylating agents. Sodium thiosulfate prevents alkylation and tissue destruction and is administered subcutaneously into the affected tissue. Hyaluronidase is known to be an effective antidote for Vinca alkaloids along with application of warm packs and elevation of the affected site. Totect is the antidote of choice for extravasation of anthracyclines. Cold compresses and topical DMSO are useful in extravasation of anti-tumor antibiotics. Ice is indicated in management of taxane extravasation.

139. C: Fatigue in cancer patients is not only the most common symptom experienced but also the most distressing. Severe fatigue in patients with advanced cancer is quite prevalent, with approximately 75% of patients experiencing it. Fatigue is often accompanied by pain, insomnia, and depression or anxiety. There are many factors that contribute to fatigue including the underlying disease, treatment, anemia, malnutrition, sleep disorders, metabolic disturbances, and depression. Fatigue is subjective and is reported by patients as a tiredness affecting the whole body, impacting the ability to perform basic tasks. It is not relieved by sleep or rest.

140. A: Increased protein degradation may occur as a metabolic change caused by malignancy. Gluconeogenesis is increased in malignancy, with an estimated 10% increase in energy expenditure. Alterations in protein metabolism occur, resulting in utilization of muscle to meet increased metabolic demands. This may cause hypoalbuminemia, an increased uptake in amino acids by tumor cells, increased protein degradation, protein loss, and a negative nitrogen balance. Patients may become cachectic despite food intake due to the loss of protein and depletion of muscle mass. Weight loss may be further enhanced by loss of appetite, alteration in taste and smell, and nausea and vomiting.

141. C: There are approximately 13.7 million cancer survivors living in the United States today, with projected growth to 18 million by the year 2020. Women make up the largest proportion of cancer survivors. Breast cancer survivors are the largest group, followed by prostate cancer and lung cancer. The majority of cancer survivors are age 65 or older. It is predicted that by the year 2020, two-thirds of cancer survivors will be over the age of 65.

142. C: Cultural competence and sensitivity is essential for all healthcare providers to possess. Understanding how culture affects health care practices and adapting the care provided to meet the cultural needs of the patient is vitally important. Specific cultural and ethnic populations carry different cancer risks, lifestyle risk factors, and barriers to prevention. Native Americans carry the lowest overall cancer incidence and mortality of all the U.S. populations.

143. C: With more and more patients accessing the Internet for health information, it is important for healthcare providers to provide guidance for navigating the Web. The most important thing to emphasize for patients seeking health information online is that not everything on the Internet is true. Patients seeking information online should verify that the creator of the website is reputable with appropriate sources or references listed. Additionally, not all websites are well maintained so ensuring the site is current is important as well. Many healthcare institutions provide a list of reputable sites for patients to access information.

144. D: Systemic inflammatory response syndrome (SIRS) is defined as the body's response to an inflammatory process. To diagnose SIRS, two or more of the following criteria must be present: temperature greater than 38 degrees or less than 36 degrees Celsius, heart rate greater than 90 beats per minute, respiratory rate greater than 20 breaths per minute, $PaCO_2$ less than 32 mmHg, white blood cell count greater than 12,000 or less than 4,000, or greater than 10% bands.

145. A: Chemotherapy can be neurotoxic, causing symptoms of weakness, neuropathies, alteration in mental status, hallucinations, decreased or absent deep tendon reflexes, footdrop, severe constipation, and paralytic ileus. The drugs most commonly associated with neurotoxicity include ifosfamide, vinblastine, vincristine, etoposide, 5-fluorouracil, high-dose and/or intrathecal administration of cytarabine, carboplatin, cisplatin and methotrexate.

146. D: Vinca plant alkaloids and taxanes. Although the exact mechanism on how chemotherapeutic agents cause joint and muscle pain is uncertain, there is an association with agents that inhibit microtubular function (the vinca plant alkaloids and the taxanes) and arthralgias and myalgias. Microtubules play a vital role in both cell division and mitosis. With both vinca alkaloids and taxanes, arthalgias and myalgias can be reduced by decreasing the dose.

147. B: The use of bone-modifying agents to prevent skeletal events including fractures and bone pain caused by bone metastases. The use of bone-modifying agents are considered standard treatment in patients with lytic bone lesions. The use of these agents can prevent skeletal fractures and bone pain caused by metastasis. Bisphosphonates inhibit osteoclast-mediated bone resorption. Patients should be educated on taking analgesics around the clock to prevent pain. According to the World Health Organization three-step analgesic ladder, adjuvant agents should be used to treat symptoms associated with pain such as

anxiety or depression. Pharmacologic management of pain should begin with non-opioid therapy and progress to the use of opioids when pain persists or increases.

148. B: Ado-trastuzumab emtansine (Kadcyla or TDM-1). Antibody drug conjugates (ADCs), otherwise known as chemolabeled antibodies, are monoclonal antibodies with an attached chemotherapeutic agent. There are 2 chemolabeled antibodies currently approved by the FDA to treat cancer. They are brentuximab vedotin (Adcetris) and ado-trastuzumab emtansine (Kadcyla or TDM-1). Ibritumomab tiuxetan is a radiolabeled monoclonal antibody. Alemtuzumab is a naked monoclonal antibody; neither drug nor radioactive material is attached to alemtuzumab. Cetuximab is a monoclonal antibody that targets the cell protein epidermal growth factor receptor.

149. A: Cytokine-release reaction. Cytokine-release reactions are caused by stimulation of the immune system. Cytokine-release reactions occur more often with the first infusion when tumor burden is at its highest. About 44% of patients receiving their first infusion of ofatumumab will have an infusion reaction. Cytotoxic reactions are either IgG or IgM mediated and are considered to be relatively rare. Hematopoietic cells are the most commonly affected. IgE-mediated reactions occur within minutes to hours of drug exposure and require a previous exposure to the drug. Adverse drug reaction is a broad term that describes any expected or unexpected negative response to a pharmacologic agent.

150. C: Grade III. A grade I reaction is defined as a mild reaction where an interruption in the infusion is not indicated, nor is intervention. A grade II reaction is defined as a need to interrupt therapy but the patient responds promptly to symptomatic treatment. Prophylactic medications are indicated for 24 hours or less. A grade III reaction is defined as a prolonged reaction that does not rapidly respond to symptomatic medication and/or a brief interruption of infusion; a recurrence of symptoms following initial improvement; hospitalization is indicated for clinical sequelae. A grade IV reaction is life-threatening and may require life-sustaining measures such as pressors or ventilation. A grade V reaction is death.

151. C: In 2006, the IOM recommended that cancer survivors receive an individualized survivorship care plan that includes guidelines for monitoring and maintaining their health. A cancer survivor is defined as anyone who has been diagnosed with cancer. Survivorship begins at diagnosis and continues for the lifetime of the patient. There are three phases of survivorship: living through, living with, and living beyond cancer. Approximately two-thirds of patients who are diagnosed with cancer are expected to live at least 5 years after diagnosis.

152. D: Cytomegalovirus increases the risk of renal cell carcinoma. Colonization of the stomach with Helicobacter pylori is a cause of gastric cancer and gastric mucosa-associated lymphoid (MALT) lymphoma. The most common risk factor for liver cancer is chronic infection with hepatitis B or C. High-risk human papillomaviruses (HPVs) account for 5% of cancers worldwide. HPV is associated with cervical, vaginal, vulvar, penile, and anal cancers. It has been hypothesized that cytomegalovirus may be associated with breast cancer and brain cancer progression; however, a confirmed link has not been established. There is no correlation between cytomegalovirus and renal cell carcinoma.

153. A: Acute promyelocytic leukemia (APL). Hemorrhage can occur in as high as 90% of patients with APL. Hematologic cancers (including the leukemias) carry a higher risk of bleeding, with thrombocytopenia as the primary hematologic risk factor. The incidence of

bleeding is much lower in solid tumors. Other risk factors include sepsis, infection, medications, low albumin, anemia, and recent bone marrow transplant.

154. C: Hypokalemia. Ibrutinib is a kinase inhibitor used in the treatment of mantle cell lymphoma. Common adverse reactions with the administration of ibrutinib for mantle cell lymphoma include thrombocytopenia (57% of patients in a clinical trial), diarrhea (51% in a clinical trial), and musculoskeletal pain (37% in a clinical trial). Electrolyte disturbances, including hypokalemia, are not commonly seen with the administration of ibrutinib.

155. A: An absolute neutrophil count of less than 500 cells/mm3 or an absolute neutrophil count of 1,000 cells/mm3 predicted to decline to less than 500 cells/mm3 over the next 48 hours. Both the Infectious Diseases Society of America (IDSA) and the National Comprehensive Cancer Network (NCCN) define febrile neutropenia as an absolute neutrophil count of less than 500 cells/mm3 or an absolute neutrophil count of 1,000 cells/mm3 predicted to decline to less than 500 cells/mm3 over the next 48 hours. Fever is defined as an oral temperature in neutropenic patients of greater than 38 degrees Celsius sustained for 1 hour or an occurrence of an oral temperature greater than 38.3 degrees Celsius.

156. D: Screening for women 21-29 years of age is recommended every 3 years. According to the American Cancer Society, the American Society for Colposcopy and Cervical Pathology (ASCCP), and the American Society for Clinical Pathology (ASCP), screening for cervical cancer (using cytology, either conventional or liquid based) for women 21-29 years of age is recommended every 3 years. Screening should begin at age 21, regardless of the age of onset of sexual activity. Recommendations for screening of women who have received the HPV vaccination are the same as those for women who have not received the vaccination.

157. D: "I will have a colonoscopy every 3 years as part of my screening for colon cancer." According to the U.S Preventive Services Task Force (USPSTF) recommendations, colon cancer screening should begin at age 50. For patients with a close relative with colorectal polyps or colorectal cancer, patients with inflammatory bowel disease, or patients with a familial adenomatous polyposis (FAP), screening may be recommended at an earlier age. Screening can be performed using high-sensitivity fecal occult blood testing (recommend yearly testing), sigmoidoscopy (recommend every 5 years or if performed in combination with high-sensitivity fecal occult blood testing every 3 years), or colonoscopy (recommend every 10 years).

158. A: Advanced or metastatic gastric or gastroesophageal junction adenocarcinoma. Ramucirumab (Cyramza) was approved by the FDA in April 2014 for the treatment of advanced or metastatic gastric or gastroesophageal junction adenocarcinoma. Ramucirumab is a recombinant monoclonal antibody that binds to vascular endothelial growth factor receptor 2 (VEGFR2) and blocks the activation of the receptor. Ramucirumab is not indicated for the treatment of renal cell carcinoma, lung cancer, or chronic lymphocytic leukemia.

159. C: Use a toothpaste with a neutral taste that contains fluoride. Soft nylon-bristled toothbrushes are recommended for use. The patient should frequently rinse his/her mouth with water or a bland rinse (saline or sodium bicarbonate solution may be used). Electric toothbrushes should only be used if they do not cause trauma. Toothpastes containing

- 55 -

fluoride are recommended. Flossing is recommended once daily using a technique that minimizes trauma. Neutral-tasting toothpaste is recommended because flavoring can cause irritation to the oral cavity.

160. C: Consider the use of a sialogogue to increase salivary flow. A reduction in chewing or mastication contributes to the atrophy of salivary glands and can worsen xerostomia. Gum or hard candy can help to stimulate saliva production; however, sugar-free gums and candies should be used to prevent destruction of dental enamel and dental cavity formation. Fluoride toothpastes should be used to minimize the formation of dental cavities. Sialogogues contain the cholinergic drug pilocarpine that stimulates salivary flow.

161. C: Humanized monoclonal IgG4 antibody directed against human cell surface receptor PD-1 (programmed cell death). Pembrolizumab (Keytruda) is a humanized monoclonal IgG4 antibody directed against human cell surface receptor PD-1 (programmed cell death). It is the first PD-1 inhibitor to be granted FDA approval in the United States. Cetuximab is an example of a recombinant, chimeric monoclonal antibody directed against the epidermal growth factor (EGFR). Trastuzumab is an example of a recombinant humanized monoclonal antibody directed against the human epidermal growth factor receptor 2 (HER2). Alemtuzumab is an example of a recombinant DNA derived humanized monoclonal antibody directed against the cell surface glycoprotein CD52.

162. B: NK1 receptor antagonist. Aprepitant is a NK1 (neurokinin 1) receptor antagonist used in combination with other antiemetic agents for the prevention of acute and delayed nausea and vomiting associated with highly emetogenic cancer chemotherapy. 5HT3 receptor antagonists used to treat CINV include ondansetron, granisetron, dolasetron, and palonosetron. Dopamine receptor antagonists used to treat CINV include metoclopramide, prochlorperazine, and haloperidol. Dexamethasone is a corticosteroid that may be used to treat CINV.

163. B: Grade 2. According to the National Cancer Institute's Common Terminology Criteria for Adverse Events (CTCAE), the patient's diarrhea would be classified as a grade 2. Grade 2 diarrhea is defined as an increase of 4-6 stools/day over baseline. Grade 1 is defined as an increase of less than 4 stools per day over baseline. Grade 3 diarrhea is defined as an increase of greater than or equal to 7 stools/day over baseline. Grade 4 diarrhea is defined as life-threatening consequence; urgent intervention is needed.

164. D: Ringing in the ears. Chemotherapy-induced peripheral neuropathy can manifest in the form of sensory symptoms, motor symptoms, cranial symptoms, and autonomic symptoms. Pain, loss of sensation, numbness/tingling, burning, tripping and falling, and difficultly walking and placing feet are all sensory symptoms that a patient may experience with chemotherapy-induced peripheral neuropathy. Ringing in the ears and hoarseness are cranial symptoms that may occur with chemotherapy-induced peripheral neuropathy.

165. D: 5-Fluorouracil. Certain chemotherapeutic agents have a higher propensity for the development of peripheral neuropathy. Chemotherapeutic agents that are linked to the development of chemotherapy-induced peripheral neuropathy include platinum drugs (such as cisplatin), taxanes, epothilones, plant alkaloids (such as vincristine), thalidomide, bortezomib, and eribulin. The incidence of chemotherapy-induced peripheral neuropathy with 5-fluorouracil is low and considered rare.

Practice Test #2

Practice Questions

1. A patient receiving IV doxorubicin, an anthracycline DNA-binding agent, for breast cancer develops swelling, redness, itching, and vesicles at the IV insertion site. After discontinuing the medication, the nurse should:
    a. apply ice and administer dexrazoxane.
    b. apply a heating pad and administer dexrazoxane.
    c. apply heat and dimethyl sulfoxide to the affected tissue.
    d. inject dexamethasone into the affected tissue.

2. When a Buddhist patient dies, the family asks that no one touch the body for at least four hours. The most likely reason for this is that the family:
    a. needs time to come to terms with the patient's death.
    b. believes that the soul stays with the body after death and needs time to leave in peace.
    c. wants time to pray for the patient's soul.
    d. wants time to wash and prepare the body.

3. The nurse enters a patient's room and finds the patient shaking and distraught. He has just spoken with his doctor. What should the nurse say?
    a. "What's wrong?"
    b. "Do you want me to call your family?"
    c. "You are shaking and seem worried."
    d. "You don't need to worry. Everything will be all right."

4. A 48 year-old female patient has stage IV ovarian cancer but states that she believes her doctor has misdiagnosed her and requests to see a different doctor. Which stage of Elisabeth Kübler-Ross's stages of grief is she likely experiencing?
    a. Anger
    b. Denial
    c. Depression
    d. Bargaining

5. Which governmental agency regulates the protection of human subjects and states that when performing studies involving people, the researcher must first obtain informed consent, in easily understandable language?
    a. FDA
    b. OSHA
    c. CDC
    d. EPA

6. Which of the following is a part of formal closure activities once a patient dies?
    a. Sending a gift to the surviving family member
    b. Sending a condolence card
    c. Assisting family in making funeral arrangements
    d. Establishing an ongoing long-term relationship

7. An immunocompromised patient has developed a systemic infection. Her temperature is 39°C, and she has tachypnea, tachycardia, and leukocytosis (20,000 / mm³). Based on these symptoms, the infection would be classified as:
    a. Bacteremia
    b. Septic shock
    c. Multiorgan Dysfunction Syndrome
    d. Systemic Inflammatory Response Syndrome

8. The most common cause of lung cancer is:
    a. A genetic mutation
    b. Exposure to smog
    c. Exposure to direct or secondary tobacco smoke
    d. Exposure to industrial chemicals

9. A hospice patient nearing death should be offered food and fluids until:
    a. The patient loses consciousness.
    b. The patient stops showing interest in eating or drinking.
    c. The patient begins artificial feeding and hydration.
    d. The patient becomes lethargic, sleeping much of the time.

10. A patient nearing death has been experiencing delirium, with marked confusion and hallucinations. The patient believes the nurse is her child and asks if everything is all right at home. An appropriate response is:
    a. "Everything is fine at home."
    b. "You are confused about who I am."
    c. "I am your nurse, John Smith."
    d. "I'm not your child."

11. A 70 year-old male with prostate cancer complains of lower back pain and vertebral tenderness, which increases when he bears down for a bowel movement. He is also experiencing increased muscle weakness, changes in bowel function, and sensory paresthesia. The most likely cause of these symptoms is:
    a. Spinal cord compression
    b. Bowel obstruction
    c. Urinary infection
    d. Back strain

12. When applying for employment after surviving cancer, which of the following should the applicant do at the initial interview?
    a. Provide a doctor's note regarding treatment and current status.
    b. Explain in detail the type of cancer and extent of treatment.
    c. Ask if the company insurance covers any future cancer treatment.
    d. Outline personal qualifications for the job.

13. A patient taking opioids for pain management is having increased constipation and has started bowel retraining. When is the best time to assist the patient in sitting on a toilet or commode to promote bowel evacuation?
    a. When the patient first wakes up in the morning
    b. About 20 to 30 minutes after a meal
    c. When the patient feels an urge to defecate
    d. Right before bedtime

14. In which of the following ethnic groups do males have the highest risk of developing cancer?
    a. African Americans
    b. Asians
    c. Caucasians
    d. Hispanics

15. A patient dying of lung cancer is dyspneic. When the nurse goes into his room, she finds that the head of his bed is elevated to 45° and he is receiving oxygen at 4L/min. Which of the following interventions can best help the patient feel less short of breath?
    a. Playing soft music
    b. Increasing fluid intake
    c. Directing the airflow of an electric fan toward the patient's face
    d. Sitting the patient upright (at 90°) in bed

16. A patient has had persistent nausea and vomiting, despite receiving medication to control her symptoms. Which of the following measures may provide some relief?
    a. Increasing fluid intake with meals
    b. Serving foods at a warm to hot temperature
    c. Asking the patient lie flat after eating
    d. Asking the patient to do deep breathing and controlled swallowing maneuvers

17. As a patient nears death, an audible gurgling is heard as the patient breathes. Which of the following is the best way to explain this sound to visiting family members?
    a. "Congestion in the throat and lungs occurs as fluids accumulate."
    b. "These are the death rattles."
    c. "He is starting to drown in his own body fluids."
    d. "This sounds bad, but it's perfectly normal."

18. Tumor cells that have been described as undifferentiated are expected to:
    a. Behave like normal cells
    b. Grow rapidly
    c. Remain in situ
    d. Grow slowly

19. As a patient is nearing death, the patient's daughter states that she would like to do something to help care for her mother, but she is unsure what to do. The nurse should:
    a. Tell the daughter that her presence is enough.
    b. Tell the daughter her help isn't needed.
    c. Tell the daughter to hold her mother's hand and talk to her.
    d. Show the daughter how to do simple procedures, such as mouth care.

20. Which of the following describes the primary purpose of a cancer survivorship plan?
    a. Outline options for hospice care
    b. Outline expected follow-up care after achieving remission
    c. Outline therapies received during primary treatment
    d. Outline legal issues, such as advance directives

21. What is a proto-oncogene?
    a. A gene that has the potential to become a gene that transforms a cell into a tumor cell
    b. An abnormal gene that can induce tumor growth
    c. A gene that suppresses abnormal cell growth
    d. A gene that causes a tumor cell to revert back to a normal cell

22. A gay man dying of leukemia asks that his parents, who have come to the hospice begging to see him, not be allowed into his room because they have refused to accept his lifestyle or his partner. The best action for the nurse is to:
    a. Urge the man to reconsider.
    b. Allow the parents into the room.
    c. Tell the parents that their son does not want to see them.
    d. Tell the parents they can leave a message for their son but cannot visit him.

23. When working with a patient with a terminal disease, which statement is most helpful in assisting the patient to reframe hope?
    a. "You still have time left."
    b. "Your faith is strong, and that will help you."
    c. "What is most important to you?"
    d. "We will be there to help you."

24. When developing multidisciplinary teams, what size team is most effective?
    a. 1 - 5 members
    b. 6 - 10 members
    c. 11 - 15 members
    d. 16 - 20 members

25. A patient with ovarian cancer is using Fentanyl patches to control her pain. She mentions to the nurse that she suddenly has difficulty urinating and is only able to pass small amounts of urine at a time. Her bladder is not distended, but the patient complains of bilateral pain in the flank areas. She is afebrile and her recent blood test shows slight hyperkalemia. The most likely cause is:
    a. Upper urinary tract obstruction
    b. Bladder neck obstruction
    c. Bladder infection
    d. Poor detrusor muscle tone secondary to long-term opioid use

26. A patient with lung cancer suddenly complains of acute pleuritic pain on his left side. He exhibits dyspnea, tachypnea, tachycardia, a slight cough, and decreased breath sounds over the left chest. The most likely diagnosis is:
    a. Bilateral atelectasis
    b. Pneumothorax (left-sided)
    c. Pneumonia
    d. Cardiac tamponade

27. A young man received high dose external beam radiation for lung cancer 8 weeks ago. The patient has since developed dyspnea and a non-productive cough. A chest x-ray shows a ground-glass opacification in the area of his previous radiation treatment. The most likely diagnosis is:
    a. Diffuse spread of primary malignancy
    b. Radiation pneumonitis
    c. Pulmonary edema
    d. Pneumonia

28. A patient with advanced prostate cancer has been treated with diethylstilbestrol. A common adverse effect is:
    a. Hot flashes
    b. Increased libido
    c. Gynecomastia
    d. Bone pain

29. A daughter has returned home to assist her parents after her mother becomes terminally ill. Her father disagrees with her mother's choices regarding terminal care. The daughter agrees with her father, and they apply pressure on the mother to change her mind. Under Bowen's Family Systems Theory, this is an example of:
    a. Triangle theory
    b. Projection
    c. Transmission
    d. Emotional isolation

30. The nurse is teaching her patient how to manage his patient-controlled analgesia (PCA) pump. Although the nurse explains the process at least three times, the patient continues to ask the same questions over and over again. The nurse provides a pamphlet with illustrations, but the patient barely looks at them and states he can't figure out what he needs to do. What is the nurse's next step?
    a. Suggest a different method of pain control.
    b. Arrange for someone else to manage the equipment.
    c. Allow a rest period and then start again with instructions.
    d. Allow the patient to practice with actual equipment.

31. A cancer patient has developed white lesions on her tongue and inside of her cheeks. The tissue is irritated and painful, and bleeding slightly. Which treatment is indicated?
    a. Antibiotic, such as tetracycline
    b. Artificial saliva, such as Salivart®
    c. Antifungal medication, such a Nystatin oral suspension
    d. Mucous moisturizer, such as lemon-glycerin swabs

32. The most important factor of self-determined life closure is:
    a. completion of advance directives.
    b. death in the home rather than in a hospital.
    c. request for DNR order.
    d. honoring patient's wishes regarding end-of-life care.

33. Which of the following actions should require input from all members of the multidisciplinary team?
    a. Titrating pain medications
    b. Developing the plan of care
    c. Instructing the patient in stress reduction techniques
    d. Managing skin care

34. A patient with cognitive impairment and metastatic colon cancer is receiving pain medication around the clock. The nurse notes that the patient has short periods of hyperventilation, cries out frequently, is lying rigidly with fists clenched, and is increasingly combative. The nurse should suspect:
    a. inadequate pain control.
    b. excessive sedation from pain medication.
    c. side effects of pain medication.
    d. increasing dementia.

35. A patient's son insists that he should make all decisions regarding his father's care even though the patient is alert and able to make decisions. The nurse should:
    a. inform the son that the patient has the legal right to make the decisions.
    b. inform the patient that the son insists on making decisions for him.
    c. refer the issue to the ethics committee.
    d. arrange a family meeting with the patient, the son, and healthcare providers to discuss the patient's wishes.

36. An advanced cancer patient is being cared for at home by her daughter, who states that no one else in her family understands how exhausting cooking, cleaning, and caregiving can be. The most appropriate referral is to a:
    a. caregiver support group.
    b. psychologist.
    c. meals-on-wheels program.
    d. friendly visitor program.

37. When helping a dying patient complete a life review, the best approach is to:
    a. ask yes/no questions so the patients doesn't tire.
    b. ask open-ended questions to elicit more information.
    c. direct questions to a close family member rather than patient.
    d. use a standardized questionnaire.

38. A patient's pain has been well controlled with the extended release form of morphine sulfate, but she has developed severe side effects and is being switched to an equianalgesic drug. The dosage of the new drug should start at:
    a. the equianalgesic dose.
    b. 25% above the equianalgesic dose.
    c. 10% below the equianalgesic dose.
    d. 25% to 50% below the equianalgesic dose.

39. During the intravenous administration of a chemotherapeutic agent, the patient has a sudden onset of dyspnea, wheezing, hypotension, and throat and facial edema. The nurse's initial action should be to:

    a. discontinue administration of the chemotherapeutic agent.

    b. administer oxygen.

    c. administer epinephrine.

    d. administer an antihistamine.

40. A patient has entered palliative care. She underwent treatment for leukemia that included chemotherapy. The patient's white blood count is currently 5300/mm^3 but the absolute neutrophil count is 526 /mm^3. The patient is at risk for:

    a. bleeding.

    b. thromboembolus

    c. spontaneous fracture.

    d. infection.

41. A patient with stage IV lung cancer has developed the following symptoms: progressive dyspnea; facial swelling; edema of the neck, arms, hands, and thorax; distended jugular, temporal and arm veins; visual disturbances; headache; and altered mental status. The most likely diagnosis is:

    a. Syndrome of inappropriate secretion of antidiuretic hormone (SIADH).

    b. pulmonary embolism (PE).

    c. superior vena cava syndrome (SVCS).

    d. spinal cord compression.

42. A patient with ovarian cancer suddenly develops severe nausea. She is vomiting large volumes of fluid. Her abdomen is painful and rigid on palpation, and bowel sounds are diminished. She reports feeling short of breath. She is afebrile. She reports that she has had only very small bowel movements recently. The most likely diagnosis is:

    a. fecal impaction.

    b. obstruction of small intestines.

    c. obstruction of colon.

    d. peritonitis.

43. A 25 year-old patient who has a BRCA1 mutation has recently had bilateral preventative mastectomies for breast cancer. Which other type of cancer should she be screened for every 6 months?

    a. Ovarian

    b. Lymphoma

    c. Breast

    d. Brain

44. According to the ANA Code of Ethics, the nurse's primary responsibility is to whom?

    a. The organization

    b. Herself

    c. The patient

    d. The physician

45. To prevent anticipatory nausea from chemotherapy, anti-nausea medication should be administered:
    a. Before chemotherapy treatment and for two to three days after treatment.
    b. Daily during the course of chemotherapy.
    c. When nausea occurs during the course of chemotherapy.
    d. For one week prior to chemotherapy treatment and one week after.

46. A patient receiving chemotherapy has developed oral mucositis, and the patient states that brushing her teeth with toothpaste increases her mouth pain. What should the patient use as an alternative?
    a. Standard mouthwash
    b. Water only
    c. Lidocaine-based mouthwash
    d. Salt water

47. Which of the following tests is most accurate for determining acute changes in nutritional status and to monitor dietary status for a patient with cachexia?
    a. Transferrin
    b. Total protein
    c. Albumin
    d. Prealbumin

48. A nurse is presenting to the staff about the side effects of chemotherapy. When discussing ethical principles related to the topic, the nurse points out that a good effect must have more benefit than a bad effect has harm. This relates to which of the following ethical principles?
    a. Beneficence
    b. Nonmaleficence
    c. Autonomy
    d. Justice

49. Which of the following is a core concept of Continuous Quality Improvement (CQI)?
    a. Problems relate to processes and variations in process, lead to variations in results.
    b. Change emanates from the top.
    c. Process improvement must be systemic to be successful.
    d. Organizational transparency must be instituted.

50. A 20 year-old survivor of childhood brain cancer is now complaining of fatigue, weight gain, muscle weakness, dysmenorrhea, and depression. She underwent surgery and radiation therapy as treatment for her cancer fifteen years ago. Which of the following late effects is she probably experiencing?
    a. Cardiomyopathy
    b. Resurgence of cancer
    c. Hypothyroidism
    d. Anemia

51. A child who was treated with anthracyclines should be especially monitored throughout life for which late effect?
    a. Cardiac disease
    b. Endocrine disease
    c. Pulmonary disease
    d. Hematologic disease

52. Which of the following procedures puts patients most at risk for development of arm edema following surgery for the removal of breast cancer.
    a. Sentinel node biopsy
    b. Axillary lymph node dissection (ALND)
    c. Axillary sampling
    d. Axillary radiation therapy

53. Which of the following actions by a cancer survivor's employer (12 employee company) is considered discrimination under the Americans with Disabilities Act (ADA)?
    a. The employer asks if the patient requires accommodations.
    b. The employer denies the patient's request for unpaid medical leave.
    c. The employer refuses to retrain the patient, who can no longer carry out the major duties required by the position.
    d. The employer requires that the patient complete cognitive ability testing because of his cancer diagnosis.

54. A 15 year-old male patient is to undergo chemotherapy and radiation, which may result in impaired fertility. Which of the following is the best option?
    a. Hormonal therapy during treatment
    b. Testicular biopsy
    c. Sperm banking
    d. Wait and watch, with periodic semen analyses to detect changes in sperm count

55. A patient who has received adjuvant chemotherapy is very distressed about cognitive impairment ("chemo brain"), which is interfering with her ability to work. Which of the following techniques is likely to be most helpful initially?
    a. Maintain a detailed daily planner.
    b. Practice brain exercises.
    c. Set up an exercise regimen.
    d. Keep a diary of memory problems.

56. A young woman with breast cancer is about to receive her first chemotherapy treatment when she begins to cry, stating, "I don't think I can do this." The nurse's first priority is to:
    a. reassure the patient.
    b. allow the patient to express her feelings.
    c. complete the treatment.
    d. notify the physician that the treatment must be delayed.

57. Under the TNM staging system, a tumor is staged T3 N2 MX. What does MX mean?
    a. No distant metastasis of the tumor
    b. One distant site of metastasis
    c. Multiple metastases far from the initial tumor
    d. Distant metastasis cannot be evaluated

58. A patient is to begin treatment with Zometa for bone metastasis. Which laboratory tests or test is indicated prior to each dose of treatment?
    a. CBC
    b. Serum creatinine/creatinine clearance
    c. Carcinoembryonic antigen (CEA)
    d. Liver function tests

59. Which of the following strategies is a patient using when she wears makeup and a wig to conceal her altered appearance after chemotherapy?
    a. Problem-focused
    b. Emotion-focused
    c. Avoidant
    d. Non-avoidant

60. Which of the following is the most common form of colorectal cancer?
    a. Sarcoma
    b. Carcinoids
    c. Adenocarcinoma
    d. Melanoma

61. Considering the stages of professional role transition during the first 12 months of a new job, what stage is the nurse going through when a transition crisis occurs?
    a. Doing (stage 1)
    b. Being (stage 2)
    c. Knowing (stage 3)
    d. Evaluation (stage 4)

62. What is the primary purpose of hyperfractionation of radiotherapy for head and neck tumors?
    a. To reduce the time needed for therapy.
    b. To reduce adverse effects of prolonged therapy.
    c. To attack cancer cells that are regenerating at a slower rate.
    d. To attack cancer cells that are regenerating at a faster rate.

63. What is the most common treatment for thrombotic thrombocytopenic purpura (TTP)?
    a. Plasma exchange
    b. Corticosteroids
    c. Platelet transfusion
    d. Transfusion of packed red blood cells

64. According to Knowles' theory of andragogy, which of the following characteristics applies to adult learners?
    a. They require direction.
    b. They are unmotivated.
    c. They are more concerned with relevancy.
    d. They are impractical.

65. When performing research studies, what is the purpose of risk stratification?
   a. To predict risk factors.
   b. To eliminate risk factors.
   c. To account for confounding and differences in risk factors.
   d. To account for co-morbidities in target populations.

66. A patient develops tumor lysis syndrome within 24 hours of initiation of chemotherapy for lymphoma. The primary goals of treating tumor lysis syndrome are to:
   a. increase urine production and decrease uric acid concentration.
   b. decrease infection and prevent shock.
   c. prevent hemorrhage and shock.
   d. decrease infection and urine production.

67. An Hmong patient with fourth stage ovarian cancer is dying, but tells the nurse that a shaman is coming to provide a healing treatment, which she believes may cure her. The best response for the nurse is:
   a. "That is not realistic in your condition."
   b. "If you believe, then a cure is possible."
   c. "You will need your doctor's permission."
   d. "What can I do to help?"

68. Beck's triad (increased central venous pressure with distended jugular veins, muffled heart sounds, and hypotension) is characteristic of:
   a. pulmonary edema.
   b. pneumonitis.
   c. cardiac tamponade.
   d. superior vena cava syndrome.

69. Which of the following symptoms is associated with hypercalcemia?
   a. Hypotonicity and bradycardia
   b. Tetany and tingling of the extremities
   c. Ventricular tachycardia
   d. Altered mental status

70. A patient with small-cell carcinoma of the lung is complaining of weight gain, increasing weakness, anorexia, and nausea. Family members report that she seems different, like her personality has changed. The most likely cause of these symptoms is:
   a. hypothyroidism.
   b. syndrome of inappropriate antidiuretic hormone (SIADH).
   c. metastatic brain tumor.
   d. hypocalcemia.

71. An immunocompromised patient has developed septic shock after a urinary tract infection. The patient is at increased risk for:
   a. metabolic acidosis.
   b. metabolic alkalosis.
   c. respiratory acidosis.
   d. respiratory alkalosis.

72. A patient with a tumor that has invaded the serous lining of the peritoneum has developed third space syndrome. Which of the following is an initial symptom that indicates this condition?
  a. Hypertension, decreased urinary output, and tachycardia
  b. Hypertension, increased urinary output, bradycardia
  c. Hypotension, decreased urinary output, tachycardia
  d. Hypotension, increased urinary output, and tachycardia

73. Which of the following groups of chemotherapeutic agents is cell cycle specific?
  a. Alkylating agents
  b. Antitumor antibiotics
  c. Hormonal agents
  d. Antimetabolites

74. How do monoclonal antibodies, such as rituximab and alemtuzumab, act to treat leukemia?
  a. By entering cells and disrupting cell function.
  b. They target specific antigens on B- or T-lymphocyte cancer cells.
  c. They target blood vessels that supply nutrients to the cancer cells.
  d. They alter DNA structure.

75. At what age should a person whose father died of colorectal cancer begin routine colorectal screening?
  a. 25
  b. 30
  c. 40
  d. 50

76. The most common sites for metastasis from bladder cancer are to:
  a. Adrenal glands, bone, brain, liver, lung
  b. Bone, brain, liver, lung
  c. Liver, lung, peritoneum
  d. Bone, liver, lung

77. During administration of a platinum compound for advanced bowel cancer, the patient should be monitored carefully for which of the following?
  a. Bowel obstruction
  b. Rhinitis
  c. Hypersensitivity reaction
  d. Pericarditis-myocarditis syndrome

78. A patient with a brain tumor experiences a seizure with loss of consciousness. When evaluated at 10 minutes post seizure using the Glasgow coma scale, the patient scores 12. How is the patient classified based on this result?
  a. Comatose
  b. Severe brain injury
  c. Moderate brain injury
  d. Mild brain injury

79. During which phase of clinical trials is a drug evaluated for safety, appropriate dosage, and adverse effects?
   a. Phase I
   b. Phase II
   c. Phase III
   d. Phase IV

80. Cushing's triad (increasing systolic pressures with widened pulse pressure, bradycardia, and decreased rate of respirations) is indicative of which of the following?
   a. Cardiac tamponade
   b. Increasing intracranial pressure
   c. Congestive heart failure
   d. Radiation pneumonitis

81. Which classification system is commonly used for astrocytomas and glioblastomas of the brain and central nervous system?
   a. TNM
   b. Ann Arbor
   c. Summary classification
   d. WHO classification system

82. Using the standard staging system, a colon cancer that has spread to the muscle layer and the serosa, and has invaded adjacent tissue but not yet spread to the lymph nodes, would be staged as:
   a. Stage I
   b. Stage II
   c. Stage III
   d. Stage IV

83. A 20 year-old patient has enlarged right cervical lymph nodes and has not responded to an initial course of antibiotics. Which test is indicated next to confirm suspected Hodgkin's disease?
   a. CT scan
   b. Fine needle aspiration (FNA)
   c. Bone marrow aspiration
   d. Excisional or incisional biopsy of the lymph nodes

84. Which of the following occurs during the initiation stage of carcinogenesis?
   a. Genetic alterations caused by carcinogens are reversed through DNA repair mechanisms.
   b. Repeated exposure to carcinogens results in genetic mutations.
   c. Tumor suppressor genes are impaired.
   d. Cells exhibit increasing malignant behavior.

85. Which type of biopsy, used to confirm breast cancer, requires a procedure similar to a mammogram but with the patient lying prone?
   a. Fine needle aspiration
   b. Stereotactic core biopsy
   c. Needle (wire) localization biopsy
   d. Vacuum-assisted biopsy

86. When a breast tumor is classified as triple-negative, which of the following is correct?
    a. The tumor should respond to drugs that target estrogen receptors.
    b. The tumor should respond to drugs that target the HER2/neu protein.
    c. The tumor should respond to drugs that target progesterone receptors.
    d. The tumor should not respond to drugs that target estrogen/progesterone receptors or the HER2/neu protein.

87. Which of the following tests is most specific when used to confirm a diagnosis of disseminated intravascular coagulation?
    a. A CBC with differential
    b. D-dimer and FDP assay
    c. Platelet count
    d. Fibrinogen level

88. What type of mastectomy involves the removal of the breast and lymph nodes but not the chest muscle?
    a. Radical mastectomy
    b. Simple mastectomy
    c. Partial mastectomy
    d. Modified radical mastectomy

89. A 40 year-old male who received treatment for Hodgkin's lymphoma at age 18 presents with complaints of weight loss, fatigue, persistent stomach pain, nausea and vomiting, abdominal distention, and heartburn. He should be evaluated for:
    a. Stomach cancer
    b. GERD
    c. Stomach ulcers
    d. Liver cancer

90. A person who worked with asbestos for many years is most at risk for which type of cancer?
    a. Lung cancer
    b. Leukemia
    c. Mesothelioma
    d. Throat cancer

91. At what age are women often advised that they no longer require routine screening for cervical cancer?
    a. 50
    b. 65
    c. 70
    d. Women should always be screened for cervical cancer.

92. A bedridden patient with advanced liver cancer has had right abdominal pain but is now complaining that the pain has spread to his right shoulder. The most likely cause is:
    a. improper positioning.
    b. bony metastasis.
    c. a pulled muscle.
    d. referred pain.

93. When is the most effective preventive measure that women can take to protect them from human papilloma virus (HPV) infection?
    a. Regular use of condoms
    b. HPV vaccine
    c. Abstinence education
    d. Use of a diaphragm

94. Providing all patients with literature about the dangers of smoking, the steps to quitting, and the recommendation that all patients stop smoking, is an example of what type of preventive measure?
    a. Primary
    b. Secondary
    c. Tertiary
    d. Quaternary

95. Which of the following chemotherapeutic agents is associated with sensorineural hearing loss and requires audiometric testing?
    a. Methotrexate
    b. Adriamycin
    c. Cisplatin
    d. Steroids

96. As it relates to skin cancer prevention, what is the maximum amount of time a person should be exposed to direct sunlight each day?
    a. 10 minutes
    b. 20 minutes
    c. 30 minutes
    d. 60 minutes

97. Following treatment for cancer, what is the most pressing issue for most patients?
    a. Fatigue
    b. Finances
    c. Self image
    d. Social relationships

98. Six months after treatment for colorectal cancer, a patient with a colostomy states she feels ashamed and avoids social contact. Which of the following is likely the best resource for this patient?
    a. Psychologist
    b. Occupational therapist
    c. Online ostomy message board
    d. Ostomy support group

99. According to Bridge's transition process of loss, which of the following does the patient experience in the ending stage?
    a. Re-engagement with society
    b. Disengagement from friends and family
    c. Darkness and confusion
    d. A new identity

100. A hospice nurse who spends a lot of time caring for dying patients often experiences which type of grief?
    a. Healthy
    b. Complicated
    c. Disenfranchised
    d. Anticipatory

101. What is meant by "normalizing" grief?
    a. Moving past grief to normal functioning.
    b. Explaining to surviving family members that grief experiences are normal.
    c. Receiving psychotherapy to deal with grief.
    d. Learning about different methods to cope with grief.

102. A patient dying from cancer is at home, being cared for by two daughters who have no healthcare experience. Which of the following is the most critical role for the hospice nurse who visits twice weekly?
    a. Provide medical evaluation of the patient.
    b. Report patient's condition to the physician.
    c. Provide information about community resources.
    d. Provide anticipatory guidance to the family.

103. In the United States, which high-risk behavior poses the greatest risk for the development of liver cancer?
    a. Smoking
    b. Alcoholism
    c. Drug addiction (heroin, cocaine, methamphetamines)
    d. Sexual promiscuity

104. The primary use for colony-stimulating factors (CSF) in the treatment of cancer is to:
    a. stimulate the production and growth of lymphocytes.
    b. interfere with cancer cell growth.
    c. stimulate production of blood cells in the bone marrow.
    d. aid in the diagnosis of specific types of cancer.

105. Which of the following resources provides the most comprehensive information about all types of cancer, including data about current clinical trials and research, for both patients and healthcare practitioners?
    a. National Cancer Institute
    b. American Cancer Society
    c. American Institute for Cancer Research
    d. Cancer Care

106. The most common site for metastasis from breast cancer is:
    a. the brain.
    b. the lungs.
    c. the bones.
    d. the liver.

107. Following a left lobectomy for lung cancer, the nurse anticipates that she should avoid positioning the patient:

    a. with his head elevated.

    b. on the operative side.

    c. on his back.

    d. on the non-operative side.

108. Following the completion of a course of chemotherapy for non-small cell lung cancer (NSCLC), a patient is to receive maintenance treatment with erlotinib (Tarceva®), an EGFR inhibitor. The patient should be advised to expect which of the following?

    a. Rash

    b. Anemia

    c. Constipation

    d. Weight gain

109. When developing evidence-based practice policies based on quantitative research, which of the following research methods can be included?

    a. Randomized experiments

    b. Case studies

    c. Ethnographic studies

    d. Phenomenological studies

110. A patient states that she is afraid to bother her physician with questions, so the nurse helps her to prepare a written list of questions, which she then gives to the physician. This is an example of:

    a. collaboration.

    b. team work.

    c. patient advocacy.

    d. her professional duties.

111. According to standards set by the Joint Commission, prior to administering chemotherapy, the nurse should always:

    a. Verify identification using two identifiers.

    b. Check the patient's ID bracelet.

    c. Ask the patient his/her name.

    d. Ask the patient his/her doctor's name.

112. The nurse is preparing written materials with suggestions on how to deal with the adverse effects of chemotherapy. The materials are for patients who vary in age and education. What reading level is appropriate for the materials?

    a. Third grade

    b. Sixth grade

    c. Tenth grade

    d. Twelfth grade

113. Based on results from a Pap smear and cervical biopsy, a young woman is diagnosed with stage IA1 cervical cancer (minimal stromal invasion). The nurse anticipates the treatment of choice will be:
    a. laser surgery.
    b. cryosurgery.
    c. external beam pelvic radiation.
    d. conization or simple hysterectomy.

114. What is the primary purpose of having a radical vaginal trachelectomy for cervical cancer, rather than a hysterectomy?
    a. There is a lower incidence of cancer recurrence.
    b. It is a less invasive procedure.
    c. The woman is still able to conceive and carry a pregnancy.
    d. Surgeon and/or patient preference.

115. A patient is very anxious during her chemotherapy treatment. Which alternative or complementary therapy may be most helpful to reduce anxiety?
    a. Visualization
    b. Magnet therapy
    c. Aromatherapy
    d. Therapeutic touch

116. The nurse is preparing to administer packed red blood cells (PRBCs) to a patient undergoing induction for leukemia. What is the maximum amount of time that can elapse once the cells have been removed from refrigeration, before it is unsafe to administer the transfusion?
    a. 10 minutes
    b. 30 minutes
    c. 60 minutes
    d. 90 minutes

117. A 4 year-old child with trisomy 21 (Down syndrome) has T-cell acute lymphocytic leukemia (ALL). The nurse anticipates that the child's duration of treatment from the start of interim maintenance will be approximately:
    a. 2 to 3 years.
    b. 2 to 8 months.
    c. 1 to 2 years.
    d. 3 to 5 years.

118. What is the usual treatment regimen for a 77 year-old male with chronic lymphocytic leukemia? His leukemia has been classified as Binet A: he does not have anemia or thrombocytopenia, and there are fewer than 3 areas of lymphoid involvement.
    a. Chemotherapy
    b. Radiation
    c. Combined chemotherapy and radiation
    d. A "wait and watch" approach

119. A young man is undergoing a syngeneic, hematopoietic stem cell transplantation (HSCT). The donor tissue is coming from:
    a. a matched, unrelated donor.
    b. a family member.
    c. the patient.
    d. an identical twin.

120. A patient with limited-stage small cell lung cancer is scheduled to have both thoracic radiation therapy and chemotherapy. What additional prophylactic therapy should the nurse anticipate?
    a. Cranial irradiation
    b. Participation in clinical studies
    c. Brachytherapy
    d. Abdominal irradiation

121. Which type of treatment is commonly used for the removal of pituitary tumors?
    a. Excisional craniotomy with a surgical opening through the skull
    b. Endoscopic trans-nasal brain surgery (ETBS)
    c. Transorbital surgery
    d. External beam radiation

122. How long can platelets be stored at room temperature?
    a. 4 hours
    b. 24 hours
    c. 5 days
    d. Indefinitely

123. The nurse is counseling a patient who is preparing to donate peripheral blood stem cells (PBSC). She should advise the patient to expect:
    a. to take steroids for a few days prior to donation.
    b. to require treatment for anemia after donation.
    c. to take granulocyte colony-stimulating factor (G-CSF) for a few days prior to donation.
    d. donating without any medical preparation.

124. Why is stereotactic radiosurgery (Gamma Knife® or Cyber Knife®) limited to treatment for small brain tumors (<4 cm)?
    a. Because the tumor is not physically removed and is instead replaced with scar tissue.
    b. Because the radiation dose is too weak.
    c. Because the radiation dose is too strong and can lead to long term neurological defect.
    d. Because adverse effects are too severe.

125. The primary treatment for advanced stage hepatocellular cancer with metastasis to the lungs is:
    a. chemotherapy.
    b. radiofrequency ablation.
    c. liver transplant.
    d. palliative care.

126. A patient has been diagnosed with stage II renal cell cancer (T2 N0 M0). The nurse anticipates the treatment of choice will be:
   a. radical nephrectomy and chemotherapy.
   b. radical nephrectomy and external beam radiation.
   c. radical nephrectomy.
   d. Chemotherapy and external beam radiation.

127. A patient wants to use alternative or complementary therapy to relieve nausea associated with chemotherapy. Which therapy should the nurse suggest?
   a. Naturopathy
   b. Acupuncture
   c. Chiropractic treatment
   d. Biofield therapy

128. A patient developed alopecia after completing chemotherapy treatment. When can the patient expect that her hair will begin to regrow?
   a. One to three weeks
   b. One to three months
   c. Four to six weeks
   d. Four to six months

129. A patient with a descending colostomy after surgery for colorectal cancer is concerned that she only has a bowel movement every 3 days. The nurse should respond by saying:
   a. "You probably need to take a stool softener."
   b. "You should begin to do daily irrigations."
   c. "Most people only have stools every 3 days with a colostomy."
   d. "Unless the stool is very hard, then every 3 days is probably normal for you."

130. Which of the following symptoms is typically associated with advanced carcinoma of the pancreatic tail?
   a. Clay-colored stools
   b. Jaundice
   c. Nausea and vomiting
   d. Abdominal and back pain

131. A patient awaiting an organ transplant has a 7:8 human leukocyte antigen (HLA) match. This means that:
   a. three complete HLA sets are matched and only one of the fourth set is matched.
   b. 70% of HLAs matches.
   c. 56 HLAs match.
   d. seven out of eight HLAs are mismatched.

132. Which of the following is the treatment of choice for local squamous cell carcinoma?
   a. Topical 5-FU 5%
   b. Systemic chemotherapy
   c. Mohs micrographic surgery
   d. Dermabrasion

133. A patient with a brain tumor exhibits changes in mood and personality, and has developed hemiparesis. The tumor is probably located in the:
    a. temporal lobe.
    b. parietal lobe.
    c. cerebellum.
    d. frontal lobe.

134. Which of the following is a risk factor associated with glioblastoma?
    a. Smoking
    b. Exposure to petrochemicals
    c. Exposure to asbestos
    d. Excessive drinking

135. A patient receiving trastuzumab (Herceptin®) for breast cancer has developed tachycardia. The nurse anticipates that the patient will require which of the following studies?
    a. Echocardiogram
    b. Stress test
    c. Angiography
    d. Cardiac CT

136. While receiving chemotherapy for cancer, a patient is usually most at risk for:
    a. hemorrhage.
    b. infection.
    c. cognitive impairment.
    d. hypersensitivity reactions.

137. A patient who underwent gastrojejunostomy for cancer of the stomach complains that he is having abdominal cramps, palpitations, nausea, and vomiting shortly after eating. The nurse anticipates that the patient needs:
    a. an ECG.
    b. an abdominal CT scan.
    c. gastrointestinal endoscopy.
    d. dietary counseling.

138. Which type of melanoma is the most aggressive form of skin cancer?
    a. Superficial spreading
    b. Lentigo-maligna
    c. Nodular
    d. Acral-lentiginous

139. A patient receiving chemotherapy has developed anemia and must increase dietary iron intake. Which of the following foods contains the highest source of iron?
    a. White meat (chicken) and fish
    b. Red meat and cooked dried beans
    c. Beets and carrots
    d. Oranges, apples, and bananas

140. A patient is to receive bleomycin sulfate as palliative treatment for testicular cancer. Which type of testing does the nurse anticipate the patient will need before beginning treatment?
   a. Cardiac assessment
   b. Liver function tests
   c. Coagulation panel
   d. Pulmonary function tests

141. The cancer vaccine, Sipuleucel-T-T (Provenge®), is used to treat which of the following?
   a. Prostate cancer
   b. Ovarian cancer
   c. Lung cancer
   d. Breast cancer

142. When should a person consider getting counseling to manage complicated grief if he has isolated himself or finds himself unable to function normally?
   a. 2 months after the death of a loved one
   b. 4 months after the death of a loved one
   c. 6 months after the death of a loved one
   d. 12 months after the death of a loved one

143. A patient receiving pelvic radiation is concerned that she has lost her interest in sex. The nurse's priority intervention is to:
   a. recommend the patient see a therapist about her sexual issues.
   b. recommend the patient discuss this issue with the physician.
   c. reassure the patient that this is normal during therapy and usually resolves after treatment.
   d. reassure the patient that there are other ways to express intimacy.

144. Which of the following factors contributes to a positive prognosis a patient diagnosed with thyroid carcinoma?
   a. Being 50 years old
   b. Tumor size of 4.5 cm
   c. Having a differentiated papillary tumor
   d. Metastasis to local lymph nodes

145. A patient who requires repeated transfusions of packed red blood cells (PRBCs) is especially at risk for:
   a. thrombus formation.
   b. infection with hepatitis.
   c. iron overload.
   d. sepsis.

146. Extravasation of chemotherapy from a central venous catheter may occur with all of the following scenarios except:
   a. difficult insertion of the central venous catheter
   b. incorrect needle placement
   c. internal pinch off of the catheter
   d. use of a 10 mL syringe of fluid to flush the catheter

147. Which of the following considerations are relevant with the use of mannitol to reduce intracranial pressure and cerebral edema?
    a. Mannitol is a vesicant and care must be taken to avoid extravasation.
    b. Mannitol must be administered using a filter.
    c. Mannitol should be rapidly infused via a large peripheral vein.
    d. Mannitol is contraindicated for patients with severe heart failure.
    e. a, b, and d

148. Dyspnea in cancer patients can be caused by multiple etiologies. Which of the following best describes a patient experiencing dyspnea that is caused indirectly by their cancer?
    a. Mr. Smith, a patient with esophageal cancer who experiences dyspnea as a result of cachexia
    b. Mrs. Jones who experiences dyspnea due to a diagnosis of primary lung cancer
    c. Mr. Alexander, a patient with a diagnosis of primary liver cancer who experiences dyspnea due to ascites
    d. Mrs. Hogkiss, a lymphoma patient who experiences dyspnea due to chemotherapy-induced pulmonary toxicity

149. You are administering blood to a patient in the infusion center. Your patient begins to experience a headache, nausea, and chills. The patient has had numerous blood transfusions in the past. Which type of infusion reaction is the patient most likely experiencing?
    a. Allergic reaction
    b. Febrile reaction
    c Transfusion related acute lung injury
    d. Acute hemolytic reaction

150. Which of the following is true regarding a delayed hemolytic blood transfusion reaction?
    a. often occurs in patients who are receiving a blood product for the first time
    b. patients usually experience fever, chills, chest pain, and lower back pain during the transfusion
    c. transfused blood cells are broken down and destroyed days or weeks after the transfusion
    d. the patient's red blood cell count markedly increases after the transfusion

151. Which of the following is a risk factor for the development of chemotherapy-induced nausea and vomiting (CINV)?
    a. Older age (older than 55 years)
    b. History of emesis with pregnancy
    c. Male gender
    d. High alcohol intake

152. You are caring for a patient receiving ifosfamide for the treatment of testicular cancer. The patient reports having a sudden onset of dysuria and hematuria. What is the most likely cause for the patient's symptoms?
    a. hemorrhagic cystitis
    b. urinary tract infection
    c. radiation injury
    d. bladder spasms

153. All of the following interventions would be appropriate for the management of moderate anxiety in a patient with cancer except?
    a. symptom management
    b. herbal management
    c. cognitive behavioral techniques
    d. use of psychotropic medications

154. You are caring for a patient with lung cancer who arrives at the infusion center for treatment. He states that he has recently had a loss of appetite, headaches, mild nausea, and difficulty thinking and concentrating. He is also experiencing an increase in weakness and fatigue. Which of the following oncologic emergencies might this patient be experiencing?
    a. tumor lysis syndrome
    b. hypercalcemia
    c. syndrome of inappropriate antidiuretic hormone secretion
    d. hypokalemia

155. Which of the following is not a clinical manifestation of tumor lysis syndrome?
    a. hyperuricemia
    b. hyperphosphatemia
    c. hyperkalemia
    d. hypercalcemia

156. All of the following scales can be used to measure performance status in cancer patients except?
    a. ECOG/WHO scale
    b. Karnofsky scale
    c. Common Terminology Criteria for Adverse Events (CTCAE)
    d. Performance Status Scale for Head and Neck Cancer Patients (PSS-HN)

157. Which of the following measures should be taken prior to the utilization of palliative sedation for a patient with terminal agitation?
    a. Evaluation of the patient by the palliative care team
    b. Pharmacologic management of agitation
    c. Evaluation of patient by psychiatry
    d. All of the above

158. An example of visceral type pain a cancer patient may experience is:
    a. bone pain from metastasis
    b. arthralgia from hormone therapy
    c. pain caused by ascites due to liver metastasis
    d. mucositis due to radiation therapy

159. Allodynia is a characteristic used to describe pain. Which of the following best describes allodynia?
    a. A patient that states it is painful to brush her hair.
    b. A patient describes feeling as if their scalp is "on fire"
    c. A patient describes severe generalized pain "everywhere" after opioid discontinuation
    d. A patient experiencing prolonged pain.

160. All of the following are potential risk factors in the development of secondary or acquired lymphedema in the oncology patient except:
    a. extent of surgery or nodal dissection
    b. larger size of radiation field and/or dose
    c. obesity
    d. family history of lymphedema

161. Which of the following is true regarding cancer-related fatigue?
    a. It is experienced by cancer patients during the treatment phase of their disease.
    b. Cancer-related fatigue should be measured by objective criteria.
    c. Patients report cancer-related fatigue to be the most common and distressing symptom experienced during treatment.
    d. Cancer-related fatigue is usually well managed in patients who report it.

162. You are caring for a patient admitted to the oncology unit with new-onset localized back pain. The patient is currently undergoing treatment for prostate cancer. The patient tells you that he needs to use the restroom. As you assist him to the restroom you notice that the patient's gait is unsteady and he appears to be shuffling his feet when ambulating. He tells you that he has been experiencing numbness and tingling in his feet and legs, making it difficult to walk. When you arrive at the restroom the patient states he may need some time to try and urinate as he has been experiencing urinary hesitancy. Which of the following actions are most appropriate to take next?
    a. Notify the patient's oncologist of the patient's symptoms as the patient may be experiencing a spinal cord compression.
    b. Notify the patient's oncologist of the patient's pain and urinary symptoms. The patient most likely has a bone metastasis from the prostate cancer.
    c. Place the patient on bedrest due to his unsteady gait
    d. Notify the patient's oncologist that the patient is experiencing peripheral neuropathy from his prostate cancer treatment.

163. Which of the following interventions would be appropriate in the treatment of an anthracycline extravasation?
    a. administration of sodium thiosulfate
    b. application of heat to the affected area
    c. administration of dexrazoxane
    d. flush the IV line with normal saline

164. Which of the following chemotherapeutic agents is not considered a vesicant?
    a. Doxorubicin
    b. Vinblastine
    c. Mitomycin
    d. Methotrexate

165. You are caring for a patient who is at risk for developing radiation-induced dermatitis. Which of the following indicates the patient understands the prevention strategies you reviewed with him?
    a. "I should use a moisturizer daily that contains lanolin."
    b. "I can use heating pads or ice packs for comfort."
    c. "I should avoid sun exposure and use sunscreen with an SPF of at least 30."
    d. "It is OK for me to shave with a regular razor over the radiated area."

Answers and Explanations

1. A: Vesicants, such as anthracyclines, cause local tissue damage and necrosis so the medication must be stopped as soon as any signs of extravasation occur. Cold compresses should be applied to minimize the spread of the agent into surrounding tissues. The cold pack should be applied for 20 minutes at least four times daily for three days. The FDA has approved the drug dexrazoxane specifically for anthracycline extravasation. It should be administered IV within six hours of extravasation with repeat administration on days two and three.

2. B: Because Buddhists believe that the soul stays with the body for some time after death, family members may wish to leave the deceased undisturbed for a period of time to allow the soul time to leave the body in peace. Buddhists believe that the soul experiences multiple lifetimes to learn necessary lessons and that actions in a previous lifetime influence the current life and that death is a natural part of the transition from one life to another.

3. C: "You are shaking and seem worried" acknowledges what the patient is feeling and leaves an opening for him to discuss his feelings if he wishes. "What's wrong?" requires a direct response that the patient may not feel like giving. "Do you want me to call your family" does not deal with the patient's anxiety and is an escape for the nurse. "You don't need to worry. Everything will be all right" is a platitude that has little meaning and may not, in fact, be true.

4. D: The patient is experiencing the stage of bargaining, during which patient/family may change doctors, trying to change the outcome. People grieve individually and may not go through all of the stages, but most go through at least two of them. Kübler-Ross's five stages of grief include:
- Denial — Disbelief, confusion, feeling stunned or detached, repeating questions.
- Anger — Usually directed inward (self-blame) or outward.
- Bargaining — If – then thinking. (If I go to church, then I will heal.) Trying to find a different outcome.
- Depression — Feeling sad, withdrawn, or tearful but beginning to accept loss.
- Acceptance — Resolution and acceptance of the situation.

5. A: The FDA regulates the protection of human subjects and states that when performing studies involving people, the researcher must obtain informed consent, in easily understandable language. Informed consent must include:
- an explanation of the research,
- the purpose of the study,
- the expected duration of the study,
- a description off any potential risks,
- potential benefits,
- possible alternative treatments,
- compensation,
- confidentiality,

- that participation is voluntary and that the patient can discontinue participation at any time without penalty.

Informed consent must be documented by a signed, written agreement.

6. B: Telephoning family members and/or sending a card or message of condolence, not a gift, is an appropriate closure activity. Assisting the family to make funeral arrangements is outside of the expected responsibilities of the nurse. However, making a final visit with the family after a patient's death can help family find closure. In some cases, family members may want to establish long-term relationships with healthcare providers, but this can establish a dependent relationship that may prove detrimental.

7. D: Systemic inflammatory response syndrome (SIRS) is a generalized inflammatory response affecting many organ systems, and may be caused by infectious or non-infectious agents. If an infectious agent is identified or suspected, SIRS is one characteristic of sepsis. Infective agents include a wide range of bacteria and fungi, including *Streptococcus pneumoniae* and *Staphylococcus aureus.* A diagnosis of SIRS is made when two of the following are present:
- Elevated (>38°C) or subnormal rectal temperature (<36°C),
- Tachypnea or PaCO2 <32 mm Hg,
- Tachycardia,
- Leukocytosis (>12,000) or leukopenia (<4000).

8. C: Smoking is by far the most common cause of lung cancer, responsible for about 90% of cases. People who quit smoking are able to decrease their risk but not eliminate it completely, as prior lung damage may have already occurred. Smoking is also associated with a number of other cancers, including cancer of the throat, bladder, stomach, kidney, pancreas, and bone marrow. All cancer patients should be advised to stop smoking and discontinue use of tobacco in any form, including chewing tobacco.

9. B: The patient should be offered food and fluids as long as the patient shows any interest in eating or drinking. At some point in the dying process, the patient will no longer want food or fluid, or derive any pleasure from them. This occurs even though the patient may still be conscious. Lethargy does not warrant withholding food and fluids if the patient can be easily aroused from sleep. Artificial feeding and hydration is not recommended for patients who are dying because it extends suffering, although some patients and their families may choose this option.

10. C: Delirium is quite common in patients at the end of life. It is helpful for the nurse to try to help orient the patient by saying that which is true, "I am your nurse, John Smith," without pointing out that the patient is confused. Sometimes an orientation board, which may include lists of daily activities and names and pictures of family and/or caregivers may be helpful. Reducing noise and helping the patient to relax with music or massage may decrease symptoms.

11. A: Spinal cord compression occurs when tumors invade the epidural space of the spinal cord. This complication is associated with primary tumors of the breast, lung, prostate, gastrointestinal system, kidney, and skin (melanoma). Symptoms typically include lower back pain and vertebral tenderness, which increases with the Valsalva maneuver, such as when the patient tries to bear down for a bowel movement. Symptoms also include muscle

weakness, change in bowel and bladder function (resulting from autonomic dysfunction), and sensory paresthesia. Slow-growing tumors are usually treated with radiation, and fast-growing tumors are treated with surgery.

12. D: Patients should only apply for jobs that they are qualified for and should not bring up their cancer history unless there is a need for accommodations. If there is a need for accommodations, pertinent medical records could be provided for documentation purposes, but in that case, they should be provided once an offer is made. It is appropriate to ask if a position includes insurance, but asking details about coverage should be done after a job offer.

13. B: A schedule for defecation should be established, preferably at the same time each day and about 20-30 minutes after a meal. This stimulates the gastrocolic reflex that propels fecal material through the colon. In some cases, a stimulus may be provided to promote defecation. This may be enemas, suppositories, or laxatives in the beginning, but the goal is to decrease their use. Digital stimulation or hot drinks can also be used. The patient should keep a record of stool consistency and evacuation.

14. A: African American males have the highest incidence of cancer in the United States, followed by Caucasians, and Hispanics. Asian/Pacific Islanders have the lowest rates of cancer, with American Indian/Alaska Natives just behind them. Females have a lower overall incidence of cancer than males with a similar distribution among ethnic groups. Caucasian females, though, have slightly higher rates of cancer than African American females. For both males and females, African Americans and Caucasians have the highest death rates from cancer.

15. C: Directing the airflow of an electric fan toward the patient's face may make the patient feel less anxious about the shortness of breath. The patient's head is already elevated and sitting the patient straight upright in bed may further compress the diaphragm and increase the dyspnea. Oxygen is usually administered at 2 to 4 L/min. If the patient is dehydrated, increasing fluids may increase comfort but will probably not affect dyspnea because of the lung compromise associated with lung cancer.

16. D: Advising the patient to do deep breathing and controlled swallowing may help to control the gag/vomit reflex. Other measures include serving cold or room temperature foods, restricting intake of fluids during meals, and sitting or lying with head elevated for at least two hours after eating. Patients may benefit from five or six small meals per day rather than three large meals. Fluids should be sipped in small amounts throughout the day rather than drunk in a large volume.

17. A: "Congestion in the throat and lungs occurs as fluids accumulate" explains what is happening in simple but non-frightening terms. The nurse should avoid negative terms that suggest suffering, such as "drowning in his own body fluids" or "suffocating." The term "death rattles" should also be avoided. "This sounds bad, but it's perfectly normal" doesn't help explain what causes the gurgling. If gurgling is severe and distressing to the family, there are medications that may help dry secretions.

18. B: Histologic grading requires microscopic examination of cells to determine how closely they resemble normal cells. Cells that are well differentiated are similar in appearance to normal cells and tend to grow and spread slowly. Cells graded as poorly

differentiated or undifferentiated are more aggressive and tend to grow and spread more rapidly. Each type of tumor cell is graded with a different grading system, but generally the higher the grade, the more aggressive the tumor is.

19. D: The nurse should show the daughter how to do simple procedures, such as mouth care, because this responds to the daughter's specific request "to help with her mother's care." Family members often feel helpless as their loved ones are dying, so having specific tasks can help them to feel needed. While holding her mother's hand and talking to her is also good advice, it doesn't respond to the daughter's request.

20. B: The purpose of a cancer survivorship plan is to provide the patient with an outline of long-term expected follow-up care. A cancer survivorship plan should include:
- an appropriate screening schedule for the presence of early and late effects of treatments,
- a description of therapies (including chemotherapeutic agents, pathology and operative reports, and radiation summary) received so these can be easily communicated to subsequent physicians,
- any potential toxic effects from treatment.

21. A: An oncogene is one that has the potential to cause abnormal cell growth or cancer. A proto-oncogene is a gene that can become an oncogene when exposed to carcinogens or other substance that can cause gene mutations. Proto-oncogenes contain the code that makes proteins, which control cell growth and differentiation. A mutated proto-oncogene then functions as an oncogene by inducing tumors, which the tumor suppressor genes are unable to suppress.

22. D: Giving the parents an opportunity to leave a message while respecting the patient's absolute right to prevent them from visiting is probably the best action. Then, it is up to the patient to read the message or not. Families often try to make amends before someone dies, but it's impossible for the nurse to know what motivates the parents in this situation or the history that the parents and patient share.

23. C: "What is most important to you?" helps the patient to focus on their own goals while reframing hope toward something achievable. For some patients, this may be to remain pain free while others may want to spend time with family or complete a project. Once a patient can identify a goal or multiple goals, then the nurse must work with the patient and other members of the healthcare team to ensure that the patient's wishes are known and that a plan is made to help the patient achieve his or her goals.

24. A: When creating multidisciplinary teams, important elements must be considered:
- Size — Teams of fewer than 10 members are most effective.
- Skills — Team members should have complementary skills that encompass technical, problem solving, decision-making, and interpersonal-.
- Performance goals — Teams should be allowed a degree of autonomy in producing action plans for performance improvement, based on strategic goals and objectives.
- Unified approach — The teams should be created according to the model of performance improvement, but should have some flexibility in working together.
- Accountability — The team members are collectively accountable rather than individually.

25. A: Pain in the flank area and lack of bladder distention suggest that the cause of urinary retention is an upper urinary tract obstruction secondary to the spread of ovarian cancer. If the ureters are obstructed and urine is unable to drain, the patient will develop uremia, which is associated with hyperkalemia. With bladder infection or opioid-induced deficiency of detrusor muscle contractions, the bladder should fill normally and become distended, with pain usually felt in the suprapubic area.

26. B: Sudden acute unilateral pleuritic pain, dyspnea, tachypnea, tachycardia, and slight cough along with unilateral decreased breath sounds are consistent with a pneumothorax. This can occur with lung cancer as the tumor erodes through the surface of the lung. If air continues to escape, a tension pneumothorax may occur with tracheal deviation and marked hemodynamic compromise. A small pneumothorax may heal spontaneously over one to two weeks although a chest tube may be inserted for a larger pneumothorax. Tension pneumothorax requires immediate needle decompression and insertion of a chest tube.

27. B: Radiation pneumonitis occurs in up to 15% of patients receiving high dose external beam radiation to the lungs. This syndrome is characterized by increasing dyspnea and a non-productive cough; hemoptysis may occur in severe cases. Ground-glass opacification in the area of radiation is often evident on radiographs. Symptoms usually occur between the second and third months after therapy has stopped. Symptoms often recede, but the fibrocytic changes that occur remain, and may result in persistent dyspnea. In some cases, cor pulmonale and respiratory failure may eventually develop.

28. C: Gynecomastia is a common adverse effect of androgen-deprivation therapy with DES because the balance of estrogen and testosterone is impaired. DES is a synthetic estrogen that results in breast enlargement. Other androgen-deprivation methods include orchiectomy and the administration of luteinizing hormone-releasing hormone (LHRH) or other drugs that inhibit androgen production, such as aminoglutethimide. All of these treatments may result in decreased libido. Hot flashes may occur after orchiectomy. Bone pain may occur with bony metastasis but not as a direct result of DES.

29. A: The Triangle theory states that two people comprise a basic unit, but when conflict occurs, a third person is drawn into the unit for stability. A dynamic of two people supporting or other opposing the other one often results. Bowen's Family Systems Theory suggests that one must look at the person in terms of his/her family unit because a change in one person's behavior will affect the others in the family.

30. D: The patient's inability to understand oral instructions and disinterest in the illustrations suggests a kinesthetic learner. The nurse should allow the patient to handle the equipment and practice. A kinesthetic learner learns best by handling, doing, and practicing with minimal directions and maximal hands-on experience. Other learning styles include visual learners, who learn best by seeing and reading, and auditory learners, who learn best by listening and talking.

31. C: These symptoms are typical of oral candidiasis (thrush), which is common in cancer patients. Nystatin oral suspension is used to treat the condition and relieve the symptoms. If candidiasis persists or does not respond well to oral suspension or troches, then a systemic medication, such as Diflucan® may be indicated. Providing good mouth care and keeping the mucous membranes moist can help to prevent candidiasis. Dentures should be removed

- 86 -

during the night and after meals for cleansing. In some patients, the white lesions may be absent, but the tongue may be reddened and irritated.

32. D: While advanced directives and a DNR request may contribute to self-determined life closure, the most important factor is for caregivers to honor the patient's wishes regarding end-of-life care. In some cases, when a patient is no longer able to make his or her own decisions, others making medical decisions for them may be at odds with the patient's wishes or are unaware of the patient's wishes. In self-determined life closure, caregivers and healthcare providers are aware of the patients' wishes related to end-of-life care and ensure that the patients' preferences are respected.

33. B: All members of the multidisciplinary team should be involved in development of a plan of care and in major changes in the plan, but individual members of the team may assume responsibility for the more specific roles, such as titrating pain medication, skin care, and stress reduction, in which they are directly involved. In many cases, the leader of the team is a physician, but the decision-making process should be a shared exercise. Nurses who provide direct care may have more insight into patient needs than other healthcare providers with less direct contact.

34. A: The patient is exhibiting non-verbal indications of pain, according to The Pain Assessment in Advanced Dementia (PAINAD) scale:
- Respirations — Rapid and labored breathing as pain increases with short periods of hyperventilation or Cheyne-Stokes respirations.
- Vocalization — Negative in speech or speaking quietly and reluctantly, may moan or groan. As pain increases, may call out, moan or groan loudly, or cry.
- Facial expression — May appear sad or frightened, may frown or grimace, especially with activity.
- Body language — May be tense, fidgeting, pacing and as pain increases rigid, clenched fists, or lying in fetal position and increasingly combative.
- Consolability — Less distractible or consolable.

35. D: While the patient has the legal right to make decisions, family and cultural dynamics vary widely, so pointing this out to the son or informing the patient of the issue may cause conflict. A better approach is to arrange a family meeting with the son, the patient, and healthcare providers so that the patient can express opinions about who should make decisions, when it's appropriate for the son to make decisions, and what the patient ultimately wants. This is not an issue for the ethics committee.

36. A: The most appropriate referral is to a caregiver support group because these feelings are common to most caregivers. Finding a supportive group in which to voice these feelings can be therapeutic. If no local program is available, online support groups may also be helpful. While depression is common, these statements alone are not suggestive of depression, so referral to a psychologist may not be necessary. Referral to a meals-on-wheels program may help to relieve some of the caregiver's burden. Friendly visitor programs vary, but may allow the caregiver some brief periods of respite.

37. B: The best approach to a life review is to ask open-ended questions, such as "What is your earliest childhood memory?" to allow the patient the opportunity to speak freely. While family members may participate, this is primarily an exercise for dying patients to help them see the meaning in their lives. The nurse should start with questions about

childhood and then move through the person's life periods chronologically, letting the patient guide the discussion as much as possible and ending with questions that ask the patient to assess his or her life: "Is there something you'd have done differently? How would you describe your life?"

38. D: When a medication has provided good pain control but significant side effects occur, the dose of the new opioid should start at 25 to 50% below the equianalgesic dose in the event that cross-tolerant symptoms occur. Rescue doses may be given if pain breakthrough occurs. If, on the other hand, pain control was not adequate and significant side effects occurred, then opioids should be rotated at the equianalgesic dose. In either case, the patient must be monitored carefully for adverse effects.

39. A: Because these symptoms are consistent with anaphylaxis, the nurse should immediately discontinue the chemotherapeutic agent and then monitor the patient's respiratory and cardiovascular status. Epinephrine 1:000 dilution is administered subcutaneously and may be then given in continuous IV infusion if symptoms are severe. Dyspnea is treated with high-concentration of oxygen. Once the patient is stabilized, antihistamines and corticosteroids may be administered to prevent recurrence and to treat hives and edema.

40. D: While the patient's white blood count is within normal parameters, the normal absolute neutrophil count for an adult is 1800 to 7700 mm³. The risk of infection increases markedly if the absolute neutrophil count (ANC) falls below 1000 mm³. A drop in the ANC leads to neutropenia, a severe complication of chemotherapy and some diseases, such as leukemia. Neutropenia increases risk of both exogenous and endogenous infection. Patients with both neutropenia and a fever usually have an infection that could quickly become life threatening.

41. C: These symptoms are consistent with superior vena cava syndrome, which can occur with either invasion or compression of the superior vena cava. It is most commonly associated with lung cancer but can also occur with other cancers, such as breast, thymoma, and Kaposi's sarcoma. SVCS may result in cerebral anoxia, bronchial obstruction, and laryngeal edema unless promptly treated. Treatment includes radiation, chemotherapy and surgery. In terminal patients, supportive measures such as oxygen therapy, corticosteroids, and diuretics may be preferred.

42. B: These symptoms are consistent with an obstruction of the small intestines. Sudden and frequent nausea and vomiting in large volumes that occurs immediately after intake usually indicates a small bowel obstruction. An obstruction of the colon usually results in more delayed vomiting, with fecal emesis. If obstruction is partial or inoperable, dexamethasone may relieve some of the symptoms because it reduces inflammation and swelling, as well as providing relief of nausea.

43. A: Patients with the BRCA1 or BRCA 2 mutation should be screened every six months for ovarian cancer starting at age 25, using transvaginal ultrasound. They should also have serum CA125 levels checked every six months. Oral contraceptives during childbearing years may provide some protection, but patients may be advised to consider bilateral salpingo-oophorectomy after they have completed childbearing or at age 35.

44. C: The patient. Her responsibilities to the patient include the following:
- Treats all patients with respect and consideration;
- Retains primary commitment is to the patient regardless of conflicts;
- Promotes and advocates for the patient's health, safety, and rights, maintaining privacy, confidentiality, and protecting them from questionable practices or care;
- Remains responsible for own care practices and determines appropriate delegation of care;
- Retains respect for self and his/her own integrity and competence;
- Ensures the healthcare environment is conducive to providing good health care, consistent with professional and ethical values;
- Participates in education and knowledge development;
- Collaborates with others;
- Articulates values and promotes and maintains the integrity of the profession.

45. A: Anticipatory nausea and vomiting occurs when a patient becomes conditioned by episodes of nausea and vomiting and begins to associate this reaction with chemotherapy. The most effective treatment is to prevent the nausea and vomiting as much as possible. Anti-nausea medication (most commonly combinations of dexamethasone and serotonin blockers) should be taken before chemotherapy treatment and for the next 2 to 3 days after.

46. D: The patient should be advised to use a soft-bristle toothbrush and salt water (about one-half teaspoon salt in 4 cups of water) to clean the teeth and sooth the mouth. Standard mouthwash will increase irritation. Lidocaine mouthwash is swished about the mouth to reduce pain and is not appropriate to use for brushing. Patients may also find relief with ice chips or Popsicles and some may need pain medications. If these measures aren't effective, "Magic mouthwash" and Gelclair can be prescribed to relieve mouth pain.

47. D: Prealbumin (transthyretin) is most commonly monitored for acute changes in nutritional status because it has a half-life of only 2-3 days.
- Mild deficiency: 10-15mg/dL
- Moderate deficiency: 5-9 mg/dL.
- Severe deficiency: <5 mg/dL.

Prealbumin is a good measurement because it quickly decreases when nutrition is inadequate and rises quickly in response to increased protein intake. Protein intake must be adequate to maintain levels of prealbumin. Total protein and transferrin levels can be influenced by many factors, not just nutritional status. Albumin has a half-life of 18-20 days, so it is more sensitive to long-term protein deficiencies than to short-term.

48. B: Nonmaleficence is an ethical principle that means healthcare workers should provide care in a manner that does not cause direct or intentional harm to the patient. Principles of nonmaleficence include:
- The actual act must be good or morally neutral.
- The intent must be only for a good effect.
- A bad effect cannot serve as the means to get to a good effect.
- A good effect must have more benefit than a bad effect has harm.

Although some medical treatments, such as chemotherapy, have clear adverse effects, they do not cause "direct intentional harm" and are ethically acceptable.

49. A: Core concepts of CQI include:
- Problems relate to processes, and variations in process lead to variations in results;
- Quality and success is meeting or exceeding internal and external customer's needs and expectations;
- Change can be in small steps.

Steps to CQI include:
- Forming a knowledgeable team;
- Identifying and defining measures used to determine success;
- Brainstorming strategies for change;
- Plan, collect, and utilize data as part of the decision-making process;
- Test outcomes and revise or refine as needed.

50. C: Radiation of the head and neck during childhood is closely associated with late development of hypothyroidism. Risk increases with radiation dose and being female gender. Hypothyroidism occurs when the thyroid produces inadequate levels of thyroid hormones. Associated thyroid conditions may range from mild to severe myxedema. Symptoms may include chronic fatigue, menstrual disturbances, vocal hoarseness, cold intolerance, low pulse rate, weight gain, thinning hair, and thickened skin. Some dementia may occur with severe hypothyroidism.

51. A: Anthracycline treatment during childhood is closely associated with cardiotoxicity and development of heart failure, pericarditis, and cardiomyopathy, especially the latter. Onset of cardiomyopathy may be acute or may be delayed for many years and can be triggered by pregnancy or excess exertion. Risk increases when the patient received treatment at a young age and also received other chemotherapeutic agents, resulting in hypokalemia and hypomagnesemia. Females are at higher risk than males. Pericarditis and myocardial infarction are more closely related to radiation therapy.

52. B: Axillary lymph node dissection puts patients most at risk for development of arm edema, regardless of the surgical procedure. ALND may be done if the sentinel node biopsy is positive. The number of lymph nodes removed may vary, but dissection may be level I, level II, or level III (which removes all nodes and nodal tissue). Level III dissection carries the greatest risk of arm edema. Level I or level II dissection is most common with a mastectomy.

53. D: According to the ADA, discrimination occurs when people are able to carry out the major functions of their job and they are treated differently from other employees because of their disability. In this case, the employer required the patient take a test of cognitive abilities solely because of the cancer diagnosis, so this is an act of discrimination. Employers have a right to ask if a person requires accommodations and is not required to retrain employees who cannot carry out job functions. The Family and Medical Leave Act (FMLA) governs medical leave and applies to companies with 50 or more employees.

54. C: Sperm banking is the option of choice as most 15-year-old males are able to ejaculate, and studies have shown that semen quality for adolescents is no different from that of adult males. Hormonal therapy in males has not been successful in alleviating treatment-induced infertility. Testicular biopsy has been used in some cases for pre-pubertal males with the

hope that they may restore fertility at some later date, but this is a very invasive procedure. "Wait and watch" is not a viable solution because in most situations, impaired fertility isn't reversible.

55. A: While all of these techniques are valuable, maintaining a detailed daily planner may help the patient function most effectively at work. Additionally, the patient may need to make a "to-do" list and take notes with important dates or phone numbers. Brain exercises and physical exercise are both recommended to improve cognition. Patients may keep a memory diary to help determine contributing factors, such as inadequate sleep, depression, or medications. In most cases, cognitive impairment decreases within a few months after treatment stops, but it may persist indefinitely for some patients.

56. B: Virtually all patients are anxious and fearful both before and during chemotherapy, so the nurse's first priority should be to allow the patient to express her feelings. The nurse shouldn't assume what the patient is anxious about and giving her a chance to speak will help the nurse understand her concerns. In addition, giving her time to express her feelings and calm down is enough to enable her to continue with treatment. The patient should be allowed as much time as necessary and should not be coerced into beginning treatment she is not emotionally ready for.

57. D: Under the TNM staging system, X means that the element cannot be evaluated:
- Tumor (T): Staged as "X", "0" (no evidence), "IS" (in situ), or "1" to "4" (depending on size and extent).
- Nodes (N): Staged as "X", "0", or "1" to "3" (depending on number of lymph nodes or degree of spread).
- Metastasis (M): Staged as "X", "0", or "1" (for distant spread).

Thus, a tumor classified as T3 N2 MX is a large tumor with moderate lymph node involvement but degree of metastasis cannot be evaluated.

58. B: Measuring serum creatinine and creatinine clearance is indicated prior to each dose of treatment, as Zometa may cause reduced renal function. Patients should also receive calcium supplements (500 mg) and vitamin D (400 IU) daily, although treatment should be withheld if the patient has hypercalcemia. Flu-like symptoms and fever are common side effects. Some people also develop nausea and vomiting and other GI disturbances. Osteonecrosis of the jaw may develop, requiring discontinuation of therapy.

59. A: Problem-focused strategies, which focus on eliminating the difference in appearance, include wearing wigs, prosthetics, and makeup. Emotion-focused strategies include techniques to help the patient cope and express anxiety, such as though visualization and positive thinking. Avoidant strategies include avoiding social situations and contact with friends and family. Non-avoidant strategies include being open about alterations, actively seeking information, and focusing on positive aspects of treatment. One type of coping is not necessarily better than another, and individuals must find the strategy that works best for them.

60. C: Adenocarcinomas develop from epithelial tissue in adenomatous polyps and account for 90-95% of all colorectal cancers. There are two sub-types: signet ring and mucinous. Sarcomas (Leiomyosarcoma) develop from smooth muscle and account for less than 2% of colorectal cancers, but tend to be more severe, as over 50% of them metastasize. Carcinoids

are slow-growing tumors that rarely spread, are most commonly found in the rectum and account for less than 1% of colorectal cancers. Melanomas are rare tumors that usually metastasize from other parts of body and account for less than 2% of colorectal cancers.

61. B: Transition crises usually occur during the stage of Being (Stage 2). There are only 3 stages in professional role transition:

Doing (3-4 months)	The first stage involves transition shock with emotional lability and self-doubt as individuals learn new skills and recognize their limitations. Problem-solving skills are often limited because of lack of experience.
Being (4-5 months)	The second stage involves transition crisis during which knowledge increases along with self-doubt. Individuals have continued stress but increased awareness of their individual role in healthcare.
Knowing (3-4 months)	The last stage involves acceptance of the new role and recovering from some of the problems and stresses of earlier stages.

62. D: Hyperfractionation involves giving two or three doses of radiotherapy per day for a few days at the end of treatment. This is usually done because the abnormal cells in some types of tumors (such as head and neck tumors) tend to regenerate more rapidly as the tumor mass shrinks. Fractionation (giving radiation in small doses) is used because it allows normal cells to recover between treatment, and it can target abnormal cells during different phases, some of which are more sensitive to treatment than others. Additionally, radiotherapy is less effective in hypoxic conditions, and recovering abnormal cells may reoxygenate.

63. A: Plasma exchange is the most common treatment for TTP, which may be induced by chemotherapeutic agents or bone marrow transplant. During TTP, small clots begin to form, damaging platelets and resulting in a low platelet count. Anemia also occurs as red blood cells are simultaneously destroyed. This, in turn, causes increased risk of bleeding. Patients may complain of fatigue and other signs of hypoxemia, such as confusion and headache. Patients also develop bleeding and extensive bruising. TTP can be treated with steroids, but can sometimes require transfusions of RBCs and/or platelets.

64. C: Relevancy oriented. Adult learners tend to be:

Practical and goal-oriented	• Provide overviews or summaries and examples. • Use collaborative discussions with problem-solving exercises. • Remain organized with the goal in mind.
Self-directed	• Provide active involvement, asking for input. • Allow different options toward achieving the goal. • Give them responsibilities.
Knowledgeable	• Show respect for their life experiences/ education. • Validate their knowledge and ask for feedback. • Relate new material to information with which they are familiar.
Relevancy-oriented	• Explain how information will be applied. • Clearly identify objectives.
Motivated	• Provide certificates of achievement or some type of recognition for achievement

65. C: Risk stratification involves statistical adjustment to account for confounding and differences in risk factors. Confounding issues are those that confuse the data outcomes, such as trying to compare different populations, different ages, or different genders. For example, if one physician has primarily high-risk patients and the other low risk patients, the same rate of infection would suggest that the infection risks are equal. However, high risk patients are more prone to infection, so performing a risk stratification to account for this difference would show that the patients of the physician with low risk patients had a much higher risk of infection, relatively-speaking.

66. A: The primary goals of therapy for tumor lysis syndrome are to increase urine production to prevent renal failure and to decrease uric acid concentration. This is usually accomplished with the administration of allopurinol and alkalinization of the urine with IV bicarbonate to prevent renal uric acid precipitation. The urine pH should be maintained at 7 or higher. Tumor lysis syndrome occurs when intracellular contents are released from tumor cells, leading to electrolyte imbalances (hyperkalemia, hyperphosphatemia, hypocalcemia and hyperuricemia) when the kidneys are unable to excrete the large volume of metabolites.

67. D: According to the Dying Person's Bill of Rights, every patient has a right to hope and to participate in religious/spiritual experiences, so the correct response is "What can I do to help." The nurse should not state that the healing is unrealistic nor put the burden on the patient with "If you believe." Patients have a right to seek spiritual guidance and/or healing without a doctor's permission. Traditional Hmong families may shun Western medicine and rely solely on healers, while Christian Hmong may rely only on Western medicine. However, many Hmong people straddle both the traditional and Western worlds.

68. C: Cardiac tamponade occurs when fluid accumulates in the pericardial sac, causing pressure against the heart. About 50 mL of fluid normally circulates in the pericardial area to reduce friction, and a sudden increase in this volume can compress the heart. Symptoms include pressure or pain in the chest as well as dyspnea, and pulsus paradoxus >10 mm Hg (systolic blood pressure heard during exhalation but not during inhalation). Beck's triad (increased central venous pressure with distended jugular veins, muffled heart sounds, and hypotension) is characteristic of cardiac tamponade.

69. A: Calcium (Ca) is important for transmitting nerve impulses and regulating muscle contraction and relaxation, including the myocardium. Calcium also activates enzymes that stimulate chemical reactions. Calcium levels:
- Normal values: 8.2 to 10.2 mg/dL.
- Hypocalcemia: <8.2 mg/dL. Critical value: <7 mg/dL.
- Hypercalcemia: >10.2 mg/dL. Critical value: >12 mg/dL.

Hypercalcemia may be caused by malignancies. Symptoms include increasing muscle weakness with hypotonicity, anorexia, nausea and vomiting, constipation, bradycardia, and cardiac arrest. Hypercalcemic crisis carries a 50% mortality rate. Treatment involves identifying and treating the underlying cause, administration of loop diuretics, and hydrating with IV fluids.

70. B: Syndrome of inappropriate secretion of antidiuretic hormone (SIADH) is related to the hypersecretion of ADH by the posterior pituitary gland. This causes the kidneys to reabsorb fluids, resulting in fluid retention and triggering a decrease in sodium levels

(dilutional hyponatremia). Concentrated urine results. This syndrome may result from central nervous systems disorders, such as brain trauma, surgery, or tumors and occurs most frequently in lung carcinoma. Some small-cell carcinomas independently secrete ADH.

71. A: Metabolic acidosis can occur with septic shock because of hypoperfusion and the resultant anaerobic metabolism and increased production of lactic acid. Symptoms include drowsiness, dizziness, headache, coma, disorientation, seizures, flushed skin, decreased BP and hypoventilation with hypoxia.
Laboratory findings include:
- decreased serum pH;
- decreased PCO2;
- increased HCO3 (if compensated) or normal HCO3 (if uncompensated);
- urine pH <6 (if compensated)

Treatment includes obtaining blood cultures and appropriate tests to determine the cause, infusing IV fluids, and maintaining oxygen saturation at >90%.

72. C: Third space syndrome is characterized by signs of hypovolemia as fluid shifts from the vascular space to the interstitial space. These symptoms include hypotension, decreased urinary output with increased specific gravity, and tachycardia. Body weight tends to remain stable because there is no real loss of fluid, only a shift from one compartment to another. Treatment includes IV fluids, electrolytes and plasma proteins although, unless the cause is resolved, the fluid therapy may just increase third space shifting with resultant weight gain. Paracentesis may be done to relieve symptoms of peritoneal effusion.

73. D: Antimetabolites are cell cycle specific; that is, they exert their action during a specific part the cell cycle. Antimetabolites interfere with metabolites required for synthesis of RNA and DNA (S phase action). Antimetabolites include methotrexate, cytarabine, and 5-FU. Cell phases in the cell cycle include the interphase (G1 where RNA and protein synthesis occur, S where DNA synthesis occurs, and G2 where DNA synthesis completes and mitotic spindles form), the mitotic phase (M where mitosis occurs with cell division), and the resting phase (G0), where the cell is inactive.

74. B: Monoclonal antibodies (rituximab, alemtuzumab, nofetumomab) work by targeting specific antigens on the surface of B- or T-lymphocyte cancer cells, allowing the patient's immune system to destroy the cells. Naked monoclonal antibodies can boost the immune response and/or block proteins essential to cancer cell growth. Conjugated monoclonal antibodies are attached to drugs or other substances, such as radioactive particles, and deliver these substances to cancer cells directly. While adverse effects tend to be fewer than with traditional chemotherapy, monoclonal antibodies may cause flu-like symptoms, hypotension, and rash.

75. C: Age 40. Colorectal screening recommendations are as follows.
Starting screening at age 50 for people with average risk:
- Asymptomatic without risk factors.

Starting at age 40 for people with increased risk:
- Family history of colorectal cancer in first or second-degree relatives.
- Family history of genetic syndrome (FAP, HNLPCC).

- 94 -

- Adenomatous polyps in first-degree relatives before age 60.
- History of polyps or colorectal cancer.
- History of inflammatory bowel disease.

Screening tests include yearly fecal occult blood, flexible sigmoidoscopy every 5 years, double-contrast barium enema every 5 years, and colonoscopy every 10 years or as follow-up for abnormalities in other screening.

76. D: Bone, liver, lung.

Common sites for metastasis	
Bladder, thyroid cancers	Bone, liver, lung
Breast cancer	Bone, brain, liver, lung
Colorectal, ovary, pancreas, stomach cancers	Liver, lung, peritoneum.
Kidney, lung cancers	Adrenal gland, bone, brain, liver, lung
Melanoma	Bone, brain, liver, lung skin/muscle
Prostate	Adrenal gland, bone, liver, lung
Uterus	Bone, liver, lung, peritoneum, vagina.

77. C: Platinum compounds, such as cisplatin and carboplatin, are associated with the risk of a hypersensitivity reaction. A reaction may occur within a few minutes of beginning treatment or at the end of treatment. Hypersensitivity usually does not occur with the first exposure to an agent, but in some patients it may. Hypersensitivity type 1 reactions are most common—a continuum of symptoms culminating in anaphylaxis (itching, urticaria, edema, dyspnea, cardiovascular collapse). Treatment is usually corticosteroids and antihistamines.

78. C: A score of 12 indicates moderate brain injury. The Glasgow coma scale is used to evaluate the depth of a coma or altered states of consciousness. It comprises 3 parameters: eye opening response (scored 1 to 4), verbal response (scored 1 to 5), and motor response, scored 1 to 6). The scores are added and brain damage classified according to the score: comatose (3 to 8), moderate head injury (9 to 12), and mild head injury (13 to 15).

79. A: Most new drugs and therapeutic treatments are evaluated through four phases of clinical trials:
- Phase I — A drug or other treatment is evaluated for safety, appropriate dosage, and adverse effects.
- Phase II — The trial expands to include additional subjects and includes further evaluation of safety.
- Phase III — Large groups of people receive the drug or treatment while researchers collect data and monitor adverse effects, effectiveness, and compare it to other treatments.
- Phase IV — Follow-up studies conducted after FDA approval.

80. B: Increasing intracranial pressure (ICP) is a frequent complication of brain injuries, tumors, or other disorders affecting the brain. Increased ICP can indicate cerebral edema, hemorrhage, and/or obstruction of cerebrospinal fluid. Normal ICP is 0-15 mm Hg on transducer or 80-180 mm H_2O on manometer. As intracranial pressure increases, symptoms include headache, alterations in level of consciousness, restlessness, slowly

reacting or non-reacting dilated or pinpoint pupils, seizures, motor weakness, and Cushing's triad (late sign) with increased systolic pressure with widened pulse pressure, bradycardia in response to increased pressure, and decreased respirations.

81. D: The WHO grading system is used to classify brain tumors and tumors of the central nervous system. This system incorporates morphology, cytogenetics and molecular genetics, and immunologic markers to determine prognosis. The TNM grading system does not apply because there are no lymph nodes in the CNS and these tumors rarely metastasize from the CNS. Under the WHO grading system:
- Grade 1 — Low proliferative potential and usually curable by surgery.
- Grade 2 — Usually infiltrating but grow slowly. May recur after surgery.
- Grade 3 — Have infiltrative capabilities and grow rapidly.
- Grade 4 — Active and may evolve rapidly both before and after surgery.

82. B: Stage II. Under standard overall stage grouping, higher Roman numerals indicate increasingly advanced cancer:
- Stage 0 — In situ with no spread.
- Stage I — Small, localized tumors, usually treatable with surgery.
- Stage II — Tumors have spread locally to adjacent tissue and require treatment with surgery, radiation, and/or chemotherapy.
- Stage III — Tumors have spread locally and are advancing. (This stage varies according to the type of tumor). Treatment options are similar to stage II tumors.
- Stage IV — Tumors have spread to distant organs and treatment options include surgery, chemotherapy, radiation, and/or clinical trials.

83. D: An excisional or incisional biopsy, or sometimes a core biopsy, is indicated to determine if the enlarged lymph nodes are related to Hodgkin's disease. Fine needle aspiration may give a false negative and is not usually used because not enough tissue can be aspirated. CT scans from the neck to the pelvis are usually taken after a positive diagnosis to determine the spread of the disease. A PET scan may also be done to identify malignant cells. A bone marrow aspiration can be done after diagnosis to determine if the bone marrow is involved.

84. A: Carcinogenesis involves a three-stage cellular process.
- Initiation: Carcinogens cause genetic alterations in DNA, but these are usually reversed through DNA repair mechanisms, although some mutated cells may persist. However, these few cells are not usually cause for concern during the initiation stage.
- Promotion: Repeated exposure to carcinogens results in genetic mutations that persist. Suppressor genes, which prevent unnecessary cell growth, are impaired, allowing mutated cells to reproduce. Impairment of other genes prevents the death of mutated cells with damaged DNA.
- Progression: Cells exhibit increasing malignant behavior and may invade adjacent tissues.

85. B: Stereotactic core biopsy requires a procedure similar to a mammogram, but with the patient lying prone. The breast with the lesion is compressed between paddles and a series of x-rays is taken from different perspectives in order to isolate the position of the lesion. A computer program pinpoints the position, and the physician inserts a biopsy needle directly

into the lesion to aspirate a few cells. The needle position is verified by radiographic imaging.

86. D: Those with triple-negative breast cancer lack receptors for estrogen, progesterone and HER2/neu protein, so they will not respond to drugs that target these receptors. There is no targeted therapy available for triple-negative breast cancer, so these tumors are sometimes more difficult to treat and may metastasize rapidly. However, there are numerous subtypes, and some respond better than others to therapy. Triple-negative patients are at increased risk for recurrence after mastectomy and must be monitored carefully.

87. B: While a whole battery of tests are usually ordered to confirm DIC, D-dimer and FDP assay are the most specific for diagnosis. The onset of DIC may be very rapid or a slower, chronic progression depending on the cause. Symptoms include bleeding from various orifices, hypotension, shock, petechiae and purpura with extensive bleeding into the tissues. Those who develop the chronic manifestation of the disease usually have fewer acute symptoms and may slowly develop ecchymosis or bleeding wounds.

88. D: Modified radical mastectomy: This procedure removes the breast and lymph nodes but not the chest muscles. Radical mastectomy: This procedure, which removes the breast, lymph nodes, and chest muscles, is rarely done because it has more side effects and is not more effective than other surgical approaches. Partial mastectomy: This procedure removes a section (quadrantectomy) of one breast. Simple mastectomy: Only the breast is removed, leaving the lymph nodes and muscle tissue intact.

89. A: Patients who were treated for Hodgkin's lymphoma, especially before age 21, are at increased risk of developing secondary tumors (10% of patients at 20 years). The most common secondary tumors include stomach, lung, colorectal, breast, thyroid, bone, leukemia, and non-Hodgkin lymphoma. The symptoms that this man is experiencing are consistent with stomach cancer; however, stomach cancer is often advanced before symptoms become evident. The patient should be scheduled for an upper endoscopy and biopsy to confirm diagnosis.

90. C: The most common cause of mesothelioma is asbestos exposure. Mesothelioma is a malignancy of the mesothelium, which lines internal organs, with the pleura affected most often. One problem with mesothelioma is that it progresses slowly and may not occur until many years (up to 50) after exposure, making screening difficult. The first symptoms relate to the tumor site, such as pleural effusion with dyspnea, cough, and pain in the chest.

91. B: Women are advised to have yearly screening for cervical cancer from ages 21 to 65. In many cases, women who have had normal tests are no longer advised to continue screening tests after age 65, as incidence is very low. Screening includes the Pap test, which evaluates cervical cells. The HPV test, which evaluates the present of the human papillomavirus, a leading cause of cervical cancer, may be recommended for those 30 or older.

92. D: Pain in the right shoulder is a referred pain associated with liver cancer. As the cancer progresses, the liver enlarges causing pain on the right side of the abdomen initially. The enlarging liver presses on nerves beneath the diaphragm, resulting in pain that feels like it originates in the right shoulder. Liver cancer is often secondary to other cancers. However,

when liver cancer is primary, the most common sites for metastasis are the lungs, portal veins, and regional lymph nodes.

93. B: The HPV vaccine is the most effective preventive measure to protect women from HPV. Condoms may provide some protection, though diaphragms do not. Abstinence education has not proven successful. There are over 40 strains of HPV that are sexually transmitted. Some types cause genital warts (condylomata). HPV infection causes changes in the mucosa, which can lead to cervical cancer or penile cancer (if transmitted to males). Over 99% of cervical cancers are caused by HPV.

94. A: Primary prevention: Includes providing patients with educational materials and information, urging safe practices (smoking cessation), and providing immunizations. Fluoridation of the water supply is also an example of primary prevention. Secondary prevention: Includes screening for those at high risk of disease (such as diabetes, high cholesterol, and hypertension) and instituting treatment to prevent negative outcomes and progression to disease. Tertiary prevention: Includes providing proper care to prevent further complications. Quaternary prevention: Includes intervening to prevent harm caused by medical treatment.

95. C: Cisplatin, a cell cycle nonspecific platinum containing alkylating drug, is associated with bilateral sensorineural hearing loss (especially at high frequencies), so it is contraindicated with hearing impairment. All patients receiving cisplatin should have audiometric hearing tests before treatment and after each dose. It is recommended that Cisplatin not be administered if audiometric testing shows hearing acuity is outside of normal limits. Some studies have indicated that some hearing loss may be reversible.

96. B: All patients should be advised to use sunscreen and avoid excessive exposure (more than 20 minutes daily) to direct sunlight, especially between 10 AM and 2 PM. FDA guidelines advise that people use sunscreen labeled "broad spectrum," which protects against both ultraviolet A (UVA) and ultraviolet B (UBV) rays. Effective sunscreen must have a Sun Protection Factor (SPF) of greater than 15. Sunscreen should be reapplied every 2 hours. Water resistant (swimming, perspiring) sunscreen must be reapplied every 40-80 minutes (or as specified on the label).

97. A: After treatment for cancer, many patients suffer from persistent fatigue, which can continue for many months and even years, depending on the extent of treatment and the type of cancer. Patients particularly at risk for prolonged fatigue include those with Hodgkin's disease and those who had bone marrow transplants. Studies show that engaging in a regular exercise program may help to reduce chronic fatigue.

98. D: Patients who have had treatment that alters their body image, like a colostomy, often benefit from a support group for people with similar issues. While support groups vary, they usually allow for people to share experiences and support each other as well as provide information about new products/treatments. Group members may also become actively involved in outreach programs, such as pre-surgery and/or post-surgery visits to new patients, which can increase self-confidence.

99. B: Bridge's transition process of loss involves 3 stages:

Ending	The bereaved person exhibits disengagement, dis-identification, disenchantment, and disorientation.
Neutral zone	The bereaved person feels darkness and confusion and cannot make sense of the changes she/he went through in the ending stage. This is the transitional stage between the old life and its associations and the new life the person must forge.
Beginning	The bereaved person begins to re-engage and reorient, finding a new identity and new meaning in life.

100. C: Disenfranchised grief occurs when the bereaved person is not able to mourn openly because of professional, personal, or social constraints. This can occur with healthcare personnel who are expected to accept the death of patients and move on without going through the normal process of grief. It may also occur with people involved in extramarital affairs or when a person has given up a child for adoption, had an abortion, or lost a beloved pet.

101. B: Normalizing grief means to tell those grieving that what they are experiencing is normal. This is important because many survivors begin to believe that there is something wrong with them when they have difficulty functioning during a time of grief. Normal effects of grief include many different emotions (anger, denial, loneliness, depression, despair, guilt), cognitive changes (preoccupation with the deceased, difficulty thinking or concentrating, disorientation), behavioral changes (crying, withdrawing, change in sex drive, problem completing tasks), and physical effects (insomnia, hypersomnia, anorexia, trembling, palpitations, headache, chest pain, weakness, exhaustion).

102. D: While all of these are important, the most critical role is to provide anticipatory guidance to the family so that they know what to expect in caring for their parent. The changes that a person who is dying goes through can be frightening, especially to those who don't know what to expect or how to deal with them. The nurse should explain usual physical and cognitive changes related to dying and provide comfort measures. Anticipatory guidance includes normalizing the grief process for the family in anticipation of death.

103. B: All of these can increase the risk for developing liver cancer, but excessive drinking poses the greatest risk for the development of liver cancer because of the link between chronic alcoholism, cirrhosis and liver cancer. Smoking may also have an impact on liver cancer, but many people who smoke also drink, so the relationship is not clear. Sexual promiscuity increases the risk of developing hepatitis B and C, both of which can lead to liver cancer. Drug addiction that involves injection of drugs also increases risk of developing hepatitis B or C.

104. C: Colony-stimulating factors (AKA hematopoietic growth factors) are used to stimulate the bone marrow to produce blood cells in patients who are immunosuppressed due to chemotherapy or bone marrow transplant. For example, filgrastim and pegfilgrastim stimulate the production of neutrophils to increase resistance to infection. Sargramostim stimulates progenitor cells, and activates mature granulocytes and macrophages. Other colony-stimulating factors stimulate production of red blood cells and platelets. However, erythropoietin, which was commonly used to increase red blood cell production, may also increase mortality, so its use has decreased in recent years.

105. A: National Cancer Institute: Provides an A-Z listing for all types of cancer and covers a broad range of information, including genetics, statistics, preventive measures, risk factors, and treatment options as well as information about clinical trials, research, and funding. American Cancer Society: Provides education about cancer and support services for patients with cancer. It also funds research and distributes information. American Institute for Cancer Research: Promotes research on diet and prevention of cancer. Cancer Care: Provides support to patients with cancer free of cost, including counseling and support groups. Limited financial assistance is also available.

106. C: The most common site for metastasis from breast cancer is to the bones, with the most number of cancers spreading to the vertebrae, followed by the ribs, skull, and long bones (proximal portions). Bone metastasis is especially a concern with advanced and node-positive disease. Patients often experience significant pain and morbidity because of pathologic fractures and spinal cord compression. Those at high risk may be evaluated with frequent bone scans. Treatment options include chemotherapy, hormone therapy, bisphosphonates, immunotherapy, ablation, and radiotherapy. In some cases, surgery may be required to stabilize a bone.

107. D: Following a lobectomy for lung cancer, the patient is often positioned with the head of the bed elevated to 30 to 45 degrees to promote drainage, promote lung expansion, and relieve dyspnea. The patient should be turned at least every 2 hours from back to operative side to prevent pressure as well as to encourage chest tube drainage. However, the patient should avoid turning completely toward the non-operative side as this may result in a mediastinal shift.

108. A: A rash occurs in almost 50% of patients receiving erlotinib because EGFR (epidermal growth factor receptor) inhibitors affect the skin as well as cancer cells. The most common skin conditions associated with EGFRs are folliculitis (on the face, trunk, and ears), rash on the hands and feet, nail toxicity, some loss of hair, excess facial hair, and dry skin. The skin conditions indicate that the medication is working, but they can be distressing to the patient. Rash may be treated with short courses of steroids or topical antibiotics, such as clindamycin.

109. A: Evidence-based practice is based on quantitative research. Data are described in terms of numbers within a statistical format. Both randomized and non-randomized research projects may be conducted to gather information. Tools may include surveys, questionnaires, or other methods of obtaining numerical data. The researcher's role is to be objective. Case studies, ethnographic studies, and phenomenological studies, on the other hand, are examples of qualitative research.

110. C: This is an example of advocacy; the nurse working with the patient to get her questions answered. There are three levels of patient advocacy, which include:
- Level 1 — This nurse works on behalf of the patient, assesses personal values, has an awareness of patient's rights and ethical conflicts, and advocates for the patient when consistent with the nurse's personal values.
- Level 2 — This nurse advocates for the patient/family, incorporates their values into the care plan even when they differ from the nurse's, and can utilize internal resources to assist patient/family with complex decisions.

- Level 3 — This nurse advocates for patient/family despite differences in values and is able to utilize both internal and external resources to help to empower patient/family to make decisions.

111. A: The Joint Commission's International Patient Safety Goals include:
- Identifying patients correctly — 2 patient identifiers checked before administering medicine, blood, or blood products.
- Using a safety checklist before beginning surgery — Ensure correct patient, procedure, and body part.
- Improve effective communication — Establish process for taking orders/report and a read back process for verbal/telephone orders.
- Remove concentrated electrolytes from patient care units — Includes potassium.
- Pre-surgical checklist — Ensure proper documentation and that necessary equipment in working order.
- Mark the surgical site — Clear, correct, identifiable marking.
- Comply with handwashing standards — Use the CDC guidelines.
- Assess and minimize risk of falls — Prevent falls in patients who are especially at risk.

112 B: The average American reads effectively at the 6th to 8th grade level (regardless of education achieved), but many health education materials have a much more advanced readability level. Additionally, research indicates that even people with much higher reading skills learn medical and health information most effectively when the material is presented at the 6th to 8th grade readability level. Therefore, patient education materials (and consent forms) should not be written at higher than this level. There are readability index calculators available on the Internet to give an approximation of grade level for those preparing materials without expertise in reading education.

113. D: Cervical cancer staged IA1 is usually treated with conization or (most often) simple hysterectomy. Cervical cancer is staged from 0 to IV but stages I to IV each have 2 to 4 sub-stages, for a total of 11 classifications. For example, Stage IV extends beyond the pelvis or involves the mucosa of the bladder or rectum, with IVA indicating spread to adjacent pelvic organs and IVB indicating spread to distant organs. A number of different options are available for treatment at each stage.

114. C: Radical vaginal trachelectomy is a procedure that removes most or all of the cervix, contiguous parametrium, and the vaginal cuff. It leaves the uterus intact so that women are still able to conceive and carry a pregnancy. Additionally, a laparoscopic pelvic lymphadenectomy is usually completed to evaluate metastasis to the lymph nodes. This surgical option is usually reserved for women under 40 who want to be able to become pregnant and whose cancer is at an early stage.

115. A: Visualization is often used, successfully, to reduce anxiety. Basic techniques include the following:
- Sit or lie comfortably in a quiet place away from distractions, if possible.
- Concentrate on breathing while taking long slow breaths.
- Close the eyes to shut out distractions and create an image in the mind of place or situation desired.

- Concentrate on that image, such as of a favorite place or activity, engaging as many senses as possible and imaging details.
- If the mind wanders, breathe deeply and bring consciousness back to the image or concentrate on breathing for a few moments and then return to the imagery.
- End with positive imagery.

116. B: PRBC transfusions should be initiated within 30 minutes after removal from refrigeration, and the duration of administration should not exceed 4 hours. The patient should be observed continuously for the first 15 minutes of administration and then closely for at least the next 30 minutes. Any blood product that appears cloudy or different in appearance should immediately be returned to the lab. Abnormalities in color or a cloudy appearance of RBCs can indicate that hemolysis is taking place. Gas bubbles may indicate bacterial infection.

117. A: Children with ALL usually undergo a 5-phase treatment protocol: induction, consolidation, interim maintenance, delayed intensification, and maintenance. With T-cell ALL, the total duration from the start of interim maintenance usually ranges from 2 to 3 years. If relapse occurs, the child may undergo re-induction and treatment with different chemotherapeutic agents. There are 3 subtypes of ALL (L1, L2, and L3), but most (85%) of pediatric cases are L1, which corresponds to T-cell or pre-B cell. Prognosis is better for T-cell ALL than for B-cell.

118. D: Wait and watch is usually the treatment of choice for older adults with low risk of Binet A CLL with because early treatment with chemotherapy has not been proven to increase survival and may have severe side effects. Corticosteroids are often used to treat autoimmune hemolytic anemia and thrombocytopenia, which may occur. CLL is the most common type of leukemia in adults and is more common in males than females.

119. D: Syngenic: Donation is from an identical twin. Autologous: Donation is from the patient, but autologous purged transplant requires that malignant cells be removed through *ex vivo* treatment prior to transplantation so that malignant cells are not reintroduced. Allogenic: Donation is from a family member, usually a sibling. Matched unrelated donor (MUD): Donation is obtained from a donor registry from an unrelated donor who has volunteered to provide stem cells for transplant.

120. A: Prophylactic cranial irradiation (PCI) is recommended for those with both limited-stage and extensive-stage small cell lung cancer. Even if the cancer is in remission, patients have a 60% risk of developing metastasis to the CNS, usually within 3 years; PCI can reduce this risk by half. Patients with small cell lung cancer often exhibit neuropsychological impairment, but this does not seem to be exacerbated by PCI.

121. B: Endoscopic trans-nasal brain surgery, a minimally invasive technique, is a commonly used approach for the removal of pituitary tumors. The thinnest part of the skull is at the top of the nasal passage, so access is far simpler than through the top of the skull. Tumors at the base of the brain are easily accessed without going through the brain parenchyma, and previously inoperable tumors can now be removed using this technique. Because brain trauma is limited, radiation and/or chemotherapy can begin shortly after surgery.

122. C: Platelets can be stored for ≤5 days at room temperature but should be agitated before use to prevent clumping. ABO/Rh compatibility is desired but some substitutions can be made, as the number of RBCs is usually too low to cause a reaction. A person with Rh-negative blood, however, can become sensitized. Single donor platelets are preferred for people undergoing repeated platelet transfusions. Because platelets are kept at room temperature, they should be tested with rapid culturing before administration to ensure they have not become contaminated.

123. C: Donated cells for hematopoietic stem cell transplantation (HSCT) may be obtained from bone marrow (BMT), peripheral blood (PBST), or umbilical cord blood (UCBSCT). PBSCT is less invasive than BMT for the donor, but stem cells are usually sparse in the bloodstream, so the donor must take granulocyte colony-stimulating factor for a few days to increase the number of stem cells released into the bloodstream. UCBSCT is not readily available and only about 50 mL of cord blood is obtained from each donation.

124. A: Stereotactic radiosurgery (Gamma Knife® or Cyber Knife®) is limited to the treatment of small brain tumors (<4 cm) because the tumor is not physically removed as with a craniotomy. Radiation is focused precisely on the tumor, which causes the tumor to shrink and be replaced with scar tissue. Tumors die slowly—up to 2 years for benign tumors and several months for malignant tumors, which divide faster. Side effects are usually minimal, and adults can usually undergo the procedure without anesthesia. Some swelling may occur as irradiated tumor cells are unable to regulate fluids, so patients may receive a course of steroids.

125. D: While a wide variety of treatments may be used to manage advanced-stage hepatocellular cancer, the primary treatment is palliative, or to relieve pain and discomfort. Despite treatment, the prognosis is very poor with only about 5% survival rates at 5 years. Liver transplantation is not an option with diffuse lesions and metastasis; however, patients may be referred to clinical trials in the hopes of extending survival and receiving treatment that may be palliative.

126. C: Radical nephrectomy is the treatment of choice for Stage II, and Stage III renal cell cancer. Stage I renal cell cancer may be treated with partial, simple, or radical nephrectomy. Renal cancer does not respond well to systemic therapy, so chemotherapy is not usually advised, although there are some current clinical trials studying new drugs. External beam radiation does not appear to improve survival rates, although it may be used for patients with diffuse renal cell cancer. In many cases, radical nephrectomy is curative.

127. B: Acupuncture is especially effective for pain control and for relief of nausea and vomiting after radiation or chemotherapy. It can be used for many other conditions as well. Acupuncture is an integral part of traditional Chinese medicine and involves balancing Qi (vital energy) through inserting tiny needles into specific sites, referred to as acupoints, based on 12 major meridian pathways. Needles are usually left in place for 30 to 60 minutes. Specific acupoints are used to treat different organs or areas of the body.

128. B: After chemotherapy is completed, hair generally begins to regrow within one to three months although it can take up to a year for complete regrowth. When the hair regrows, it may be a different texture or even color than it was before treatment. Some drugs cause hair loss consistently (doxorubicin, cyclophosphamide, ifosfamide, and Taxol) while others only sometimes result in hair loss (carboplatin, cisplatin, dactinomycin,

etoposide, vincristine). Patients should always be advised when they are taking drugs that may result in alopecia so that they can prepare emotionally and decide how to cope with the loss.

129. D: While stools from an ascending colostomy are quite liquid, those from a descending colostomy are more normal in consistency. People who had regular bowel movements before surgery may be well controlled after surgery, but the frequency of bowel movements varies widely from two to three times a day to one every one to three days. Some people need to irrigate or even take stool softeners while others do not. It's good to try to establish a regular routine. Some people find that certain foods or drinks, or even digital stimulation, promotes emptying of the bowel.

130. D: Symptoms of carcinoma in the body or tail of the pancreas include abdominal and back pain and weight loss. Generally, pancreatic cancer is essentially asymptomatic in early stages, so it has often metastasized by the time of diagnosis. Symptoms related to cancer in the head of the pancreas are more severe than with cancer in the tail, and can include jaundice, pruritus, nausea and vomiting, clay-colored stools, weight loss, and abdominal and back pain.

131. A: Because genes are inherited from both parents, people inherit double sets of HLA (one set from each parent). Major HLAs of concern for transplant are HLA-A, HLA-B, HLA-C, and HLA-DR, so an ideal match is 8:8; that is, both sets from all four HLAs match. A 7:8 match means one set is mismatched. At one time, a 6:6 match (A, B, and DR) was considered ideal, but studies have shown that matching HLA-C is associated with better outcomes. The lower the number of matched HLAs, the greater the risk of graft *vs* host disease and rejection.

132. C: Mohs micrographic surgery has the highest rate of cure (95-99%) and is the treatment of choice for local squamous cell carcinomas. The procedure is usually done under a local anesthetic. The lesion and a margin around the lesion are removed and then examined under a microscope while the patient waits. If abnormal cells are found, then another thin layer is excised and again examined. This continues until the tissue sample is free of abnormal cells. This procedure is especially valuable for removal of lesions on the face because it allows the surgeon to save as much tissue as possible.

133. D: Symptoms vary according the location of a brain tumor. Frontal lobe: Associated with mood and personality changes and hemiparesis. Temporal lobe: Associated with lack of coordination, speech difficulties, and memory loss. Parietal lobe: Associated with sensory changes, loss of fine motor skills, and loss of half-body awareness. Cerebellum: Associated with lack of coordination and balance. Occipital lobe: Associated with vision disturbances and visual hallucinations. Brain stem: Associated with cranial nerve dysfunction, facial pain and weakness, dysphagia.

134. B: The only risk factor consistently associated with glioblastoma is exposure to petrochemicals. Glioblastomas are very aggressive tumors that occur primarily in the cerebral hemispheres, primarily in adults (especially between ages 45 and 70). They are associated with more genetic abnormalities than other brain tumors, especially alterations on chromosome 10. Glioblastomas proliferate rapidly, invading, infiltrating, and destroying surrounding brain tissue. Treatment is primarily palliative and may include surgery as well as chemotherapy and radiation. Life expectancy is usually only 1 to 2 years.

135. A: Trastuzumab (Herceptin®), a monoclonal antibody used as a targeted treatment for breast cancer, is associated with cardio toxicity. Tachycardia is often an early sign. An echocardiogram to evaluate the left ventricular fraction should be performed because the most common effect is decreased left ventricular fraction. This may progress to heart failure in some patients. Cardiotoxicity is exacerbated if trastuzumab is given with other chemotherapeutic agents, especially anthracyclines. The cardiotoxicity related to trastuzumab is usually reversible.

136. B: Because most chemotherapy damages the bone marrow, the immune system is depressed and so is the ability of the body to fight infections. The patient is therefore at increased risk of developing all types of infection: viral, bacterial, and fungal. Patients should be cautioned to use good hygiene, wash hands frequently, avoid people who are ill, and avoid crowds of people. They should also avoid children who have recently received vaccines prepared with live viruses, such as the chickenpox vaccine. They should avoid going barefoot and take care to avoid cuts and other injuries.

137. D: These symptoms are consistent with the early onset of dumping syndrome, which is common after gastric surgery especially if the pylorus is removed. The patient probably needs dietary counseling to better understand how much to eat, what type of foods to eat, and how frequently to eat, as he may need to modify his eating habits. Late onset dumping syndrome occurs up to 3 hours after eating and is characterized by hypoglycemia because a sudden increase (dumping) of carbohydrates in the small intestine results in increased insulin release.

138. C: Nodular: These are the most aggressive lesions and often invade adjacent tissue. They are usually blue-black, round, smooth, uniform, and dome-shaped nodules. Superficial spreading: This is the most common type (70%) and primarily affects the young. They spread superficially for long periods before becoming invasive. Lentigo-maligna: These are very slow growing lesions and are most common in sun-exposed areas. Acral-lentiginous: These occur in areas of the skin without hair follicles, such as the palms, soles of feet, nail beds, and mucous membranes. They spread superficially initially but may rapidly become invasive. This type is most common in Asians and African Americans.

139. B: Foods that are highest in iron include red meat and cooked dried beans, although all meat contains some iron. Shellfish is especially high in iron as is liver, nuts, dark chocolate, dark leafy green vegetables (such as spinach, kale, collard greens), and whole grains. Red blood cells contain hemoglobin (95% of mass), which carries oxygen throughout the body. The heme portion of the cell contains iron, which binds to the oxygen. Thus, anemia results in a decrease in oxygen transportation and decreased perfusion throughout the body.

140. D: Bleomycin can cause pulmonary toxicity with pneumonitis and pulmonary fibrosis, so patients who are to receive the drug should first have pulmonary function tests. The drug should be used cautiously or avoided in patients with any type of pulmonary disease. Pulmonary function should be monitored throughout the course of treatment, with chest radiographs weekly or biweekly. Bleomycin is a cell cycle phase-specific agent (affecting G2 and M phases), inhibiting DNA, RNA, and protein synthesis in susceptible cells and preventing cell division.

141. A: Sipuleucel-T (Provenge®), an autologous cellular immunotherapy, is a cancer vaccine developed from the patient's own white blood cells and is used to treat androgen independent prostate cancer without metastasis to lung, liver, or brain (although it can be used with bone or adjacent soft tissue metastases). Treatment is typically given over a 6-week period with doses administered in three intravenous infusions every two weeks. Adverse effects are typically flu-like with chills, headache, fever, and nausea.

142. A: While the grieving process varies widely, most people can resume reasonable functioning, despite persistent grief, within about 2 months. Those who remain isolated and overwhelmed by grief and unable to function may benefit from counseling to help them through the grieving process. Complicated grieving is common after a violent sudden death, (such as suicide, murder, accidental death, or the sudden death of a child) because people have not been able to undergo anticipatory grief, which can help people prepare emotionally.

143. C: Radiation to the pelvis often results in a loss of interest in sex and can cause sexual intercourse to be painful for women. The nurse's priority intervention is to reassure the patient that this is a normal response to therapy and that interest in sex often returns after therapy is completed and the tissue is less sensitive. Unless the patient is extremely upset about this issue, there is probably no need for counselling, but it can be helpful to discuss the importance of maintaining other types of intimacy.

144. C: Factors contributing to a negative prognosis include lesions greater than 4 cm, age older than 45, follicular histology, extension of the tumor, and metastasis. Papillary and follicular (both differentiated) tumors have a better prognosis than medullary and anaplastic (both undifferentiated) tumors.

145. C: Repeated transfusions of PRBCs put the patient especially at risk for iron overload. One unit of PRBCs contains 250 mg of iron, and the excess may accumulate in body organs, including the heart, liver, testes, and pancreas. The usual treatment for primary iron overload is phlebotomy, but this is contraindicated in people needing transfusions, so iron chelation therapy is indicated to prevent permanent organ damage. Chelating agents bind with iron in the blood and allow it to be more easily eliminated in stool and urine.

146. D: Use of a 10 mL syringe of fluid to flush the catheter. Extravasation can occur with both peripheral and central venous catheters. Factors that may contribute to the extravasation of chemotherapy via a central venous catheter include difficult insertion, displacement or dislodging of the needle or improper needle placement on an implanted device such as an implanted port, thrombus formation, drug precipitate, or internal pinch off of the catheter. Use of a syringe that contains at least 10 mL of fluid is always recommended for use with a central venous catheter. A lower volume syringe can generate an increase in the amount of pressure within the catheter, leading to damage and potentially extravasation.

147. E: A, B, D. Mannitol is an osmotic diuretic that may be administered to treat increased intracranial pressure (ICP) and reduce cerebral edema. Mannitol is considered a vesicant and care must be taken to avoid extravasation. It is recommended that mannitol be administered via a large peripheral vein or central vein when possible. Each dose should be given over 20 to 30 minutes as rapid infusion can cause harm to the patient. Crystals may form within the IV solution; therefore, mannitol must be administered using a filter.

Mannitol is contraindicated for patients with severe heart failure as the expansion of extracellular fluid can aggravate cardiac decompensation.

148. A: Mr. Smith, a patient with esophageal cancer who experiences dyspnea as a result of cachexia. Mr. Smith is experiencing dyspnea due to cachexia. Malnutrition, electrolyte imbalance, anorexia, and cachexia are all secondary complications of cancer that may contribute to the development of dyspnea. Mrs. Jones' primary cancer is directly causing her to experience dyspnea. Mr. Alexander's cancer is also directly causing his dyspnea due to the ascites that has developed as a result of his liver cancer. In the case of Mrs. Hogkiss, she is experiencing dyspnea caused by her cancer treatment.

149. B: Febrile reaction. Your patient is most likely experiencing a febrile reaction to the blood product. Febrile reactions are the body's response to the white blood cells in the donated blood product. Febrile reactions are more common in people that have had blood transfusions in the past. Symptoms may include fever, headache, nausea, chills, and a feeling of generalized discomfort. Allergic reactions occur when the body reacts to a substance in the blood product such as a plasma protein. Allergic reactions are the most common and usually manifest as hives and/or itching. Transfusion-related acute lung injuries tend to occur with blood products that contain more plasma (ie, fresh frozen plasma or platelets). Symptoms include shortness of breath, which can be life-threatening. Acute hemolytic reactions occur when the donor and patient's blood types do not match. The patient's antibodies then attack the transfused red blood cells causing hemolysis. Symptoms include chills, fever, chest pain, lower back pain, and nausea.

150. C: Transfused blood cells are broken down and destroyed days or weeks after the transfusion. Delayed hemolytic blood transfusion reactions occur when the body slowly attacks the non-ABO antigens on the transfused blood cells. This occurs days or weeks after the transfusion. Patients do not usually experience any symptoms. This type of reaction occurs in patients who have previously received blood products. The transfused blood cells are destroyed and the patient's red blood cell count falls.

151. B: History of emesis with pregnancy. Risk factors for the development of chemotherapy-induced nausea and vomiting (CINV) include younger age (younger than 55 years), female sex, low alcohol intake, history of chemotherapy-induced nausea and vomiting, history of emesis with pregnancy, history of motion sickness, anxiety, dose schedule, route and rate of chemotherapy administration, performance status, and the degree of emetogenicity of the chemotherapeutic agent.

152. A: Hemorrhagic cystitis. Hemorrhagic cystitis manifests as a sudden onset of dysuria and hematuria caused by damage to the bladder epithelium due to metabolite breakdown products of certain chemotherapeutic agents. Ifosfamide, cyclophosphamide, gemcitabine, dacarbazine, and temozolomide are all chemotherapeutic agents that may cause hemorrhagic cystitis. The use of mesna, a protective agent that can be used in conjunction with ifosfamide, can help to protect the urothelium and lessen the potential for hemorrhagic cystitis.

153. D: Use of psychotropic medications. Patient education, social support, symptom management, cognitive behavioral techniques (e.g., hypnosis, music therapy, guided imagery), pharmacologic management, and herbal management are all interventions that could be utilized in the management of cancer patients experiencing moderate anxiety. The

use of psychotropic medications could increase anxiety and therefore would not be useful in the management of moderate anxiety.

154. B: Hypercalcemia. Symptoms of hypercalcemia include loss of appetite, nausea and vomiting, headaches, constipation and abdominal pain, increased thirst, frequent urination, fatigue, weakness, muscle pain, changes in mental status including confusion, disorientation and difficulty thinking, and depression. Breast cancer, lung cancer, and multiple myeloma patients have a higher risk of developing hypercalcemia.

155. D: Hypercalcemia. Tumor lysis syndrome is a clinical syndrome that occurs most often in malignancies with a high proliferative rate, a large tumor burden, and/or a high sensitivity to treatment. As the rapid lysis of cells occurs, massive quantities of intracellular contents spill into the systemic circulation. Rapid tumor breakdown often leads to hyperphosphatemia, which can cause a secondary hypocalcemia. Hyperkalemia and hyperuricemia also occur with rapid tumor breakdown.

156. C: Common Terminology Criteria for Adverse Events (CTCAE). Performance status in cancer patients is evaluated to assess how patients are tolerating cancer treatment, as selection criteria for clinical trials, to evaluate the progression of illness, and to help estimate prognosis. The Eastern Cooperative Oncology Group (ECOG)/World Health Organization (WHO) performance status and Karnofsky scale are the two primary assessment tools used to evaluate performance status. The Performance Status Scale for Head and Neck Cancer Patients (PSS-HN) can be utilized to assess performance status in head and neck cancer patients. The Common Terminology Criteria for Adverse Events is a standardized grading scale used to evaluate adverse events.

157. D: All of the above. Palliative sedation is defined as the use of pharmacologic agents to provide a state of decreased consciousness with the intent of limiting suffering associated with intractable symptoms in the imminently dying patient. All available pharmacologic and psychosocial treatments should be utilized prior to the implementation of palliative sedation. Palliative care specialists should be consulted to ensure that all available treatment options have been exhausted for the intractable symptom(s).

158. C: Pain caused by ascites due to liver metastasis. Visceral pain is defined as pain that results from the activation of nociceptors of the thoracic, pelvic, or abdominal viscera. Types of visceral pain in the cancer patient may include pain caused by ascites, lymphedema, or obstruction. It may also be organ-related pain generating from the liver, pancreas, or abdominal viscera.

159. A: Allodynia is defined as a painful response to a normally innocuous stimulus, such as hair brushing or face shaving. Dysesthesia is defined as a spontaneous or evoked unpleasant and abnormal sensation. This can include burning, tingling, and the sensation of being on fire. Hyperalgesia is an increased response to a noxious stimulus. Hyperalgesia is common in opioid withdrawal. Prolonged pain after a transient stimulus is defined as persistent pain.

160. D: Family history of lymphedema. Extent of surgery or nodal dissection (the greater the surgical field and/or number of lymph nodes dissected increases the risk of lymphedema development), larger size of radiation field and/or dose, and obesity are all potential risk factors in the development of lymphedema. Genetic abnormalities or familial

history of abnormalities of the lymph system are associated with primary or idiopathic lymphedema.

161. C: Patients report cancer-related fatigue to be the most common and distressing symptom experienced during cancer treatment. It is frequently reported by patients as being unmanaged or undermanaged. Cancer fatigue is best described by the person experiencing it. Cancer-related fatigue is commonly experienced in all phases of cancer including the pretreatment phase, during treatment, and months to years after completing treatment.

162. A: Notify the patient's oncologist of the patient's symptoms as the patient may be experiencing a spinal cord compression. Back pain is the presenting complaint for the majority of patients experiencing spinal cord compression. Prostate and colon cancers are most likely to cause compression of the lumbosacral spine. Additional clinical signs include muscle weakness, unsteady gait, foot drop, paralysis, loss of bowel and bladder control, urinary retention and hesitancy, and paraplegia. Patients may experience pain, numbness and tingling in the extremities, diminished pain or temperature sensation, and sexual dysfunction.

163. C: Administration of dexrazoxane. Dexrazoxane is the antidote used in the treatment of anthracycline extravasation. Application of a cold pack to the affected area is indicated for anthracycline extravasation. Sodium thiosulfate is the antidote used for extravasation of alkylating agents. The IV line should never be flushed in an extravasation situation, as it will add additional chemotherapy into the affected area. The infusion should be immediately stopped and IV tubing disconnected from the IV device.

164. D: Methotrexate. Vesicant agents cause the most severe tissue damage by causing cellular toxicity when coming in contact with tissue. There are two categories of vesicant agents: non-DNA binding and DNA binding. Doxorubicin and mitomycin are considered DNA-binding vesicants. Vinblastine is considered a non-DNA binding agent. Methotrexate is classified as a nonirritant agent.

165. C: "I should avoid sun exposure and use sunscreen with an SPF of at least 30." Management strategies for the prevention of radiation-induced dermatitis include gentle skin washing with a mild soap and patting skin dry, use of non-alcohol, lanolin-free, fragrance-free moisturizers is optional, only electric razors should be used on treated areas, and sun exposure should be avoided. Patients should use a sunscreen with an SPF of at least 30. Application of heating pads and ice packs to treated areas is not recommended.